THE ESSENTIAL GUIDE FOR NEWLY QUALIFIED OCCUPATIONAL THERAPISTS *of related interest*

Sensory Modulation in Dementia Care
Assessment and Activities for Sensory-Enriched Care
Tina Champagne
ISBN 978 1 78592 733 1
eISBN 978 1 78450 427 4

The Core Concepts of Occupational Therapy
A Dynamic Framework for Practice
Jennifer Creek
ISBN 978 1 84905 007 4
eISBN 978 0 85700 362 1

Goal Setting and Motivation in Therapy
Engaging Children and Parents
Edited by Anne A. Poulsen, Jenny Ziviani and Monica Cuskelly
Foreword by Richard Ryan
ISBN 978 1 84905 448 5
eISBN 978 0 85700 828 2

Autism and Solution-focused Practice
Els Mattelin and Hannelore Volckaert
ISBN 978 1 78592 328 9
eISBN 978 1 78450 644 5

Music and the Social Model
An Occupational Therapist's Approach to Music with People Labelled as Having Learning Disabilities
Jane Q. Williams
ISBN 978 1 84905 306 8
eISBN 978 0 85700 636 3

Challenging Stress, Burnout and Rust-Out
Finding Balance in Busy Lives
Teena J. Clouston
ISBN 978 1 84905 406 5
eISBN 978 0 85700 786 5

Effective Self-Care and Resilience in Clinical Practice
Dealing with Stress, Compassion Fatigue and Burnout
Edited by Sarah Parry
Foreword by Paul Gilbert
ISBN 978 1 78592 070 7
eISBN 978 1 78450 331 4

Understanding Sensory Processing Disorders in Children
A Guide for Parents and Professionals
Matt Mielnick
ISBN 978 1 78592 752 2
eISBN 978 1 78450 568 4

About the Author

Christine Day is a spiritual teacher, healer, and author, and has channeled information from extraterrestrials known as Pleiadians for the past 20 years. She is seeking to assist and awaken humanity during this acknowledged time of great transformation on planet Earth. She currently resides in Grand Marais, Minnesota.

THE ESSENTIAL GUIDE FOR NEWLY QUALIFIED OCCUPATIONAL THERAPISTS

Transition to Practice

Edited by RUTH PARKER and JULIA BADGER

Forewords by Dr Theresa Baxter and Nick Pollard

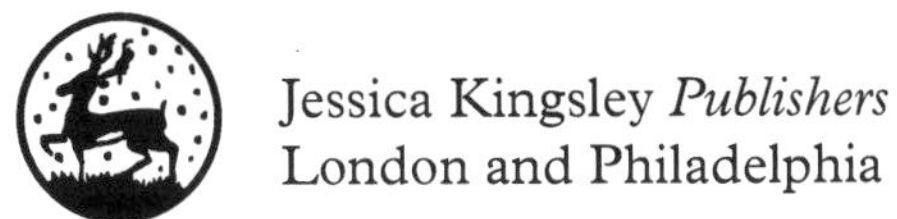

Jessica Kingsley *Publishers*
London and Philadelphia

2264 MT

The Career Development Framework: Guiding principles for occupational therapy on p.45 is reproduced with kind permission from the Royal College of Occupational Therapists (RCOT), 2017.

Figure 10.6 on pages 162–5 is reproduced with kind permission from Nigel Burton, idapt.

First published in 2018
by Jessica Kingsley Publishers
73 Collier Street
London N1 9BE, UK
and
400 Market Street, Suite 400
Philadelphia, PA 19106, USA

www.jkp.com

Front cover image source: 123RF.com

Library of Congress Cataloging in Publication Data
A CIP catalog record for this book is available from the Library of Congress

British Library Cataloguing in Publication Data
A CIP catalogue record for this book is available from the British Library

ISBN 978 1 78592 268 8
eISBN 978 1 78450 558 5

Printed and bound in the United States

Contents

Foreword

Having worked in education for many years teaching occupational therapy students, I have found that the transition to practice can be a daunting one for many graduates. No matter how much academia tries to prepare graduates for the 'real' world, nothing can truly prepare you for the realities of being a qualified autonomous professional within the busy health and social care arena.

This book sets out to ease the newly qualified professional into the working world by providing a plethora of handy tips and hints to help the graduate make a smooth transition into practice.

The initial chapter should be an essential read for all graduates; it is such a practical and down to earth guide to adapting to working life. It reiterates much of what is advised to students when they first go out on placement, such as making first impressions count and integrating into the workplace. It ends by encouraging the recently qualified practitioner to think about becoming a placement educator and passing on their knowledge and experience to others. Not only that, but to see becoming a placement educator as a great learning opportunity and to be a part of developing the skills and knowledge of the next generation of therapists. So many graduates can become disillusioned once the newness of gaining that first qualified post wears off, but the wise words in this chapter and those woven throughout the whole text will support and encourage the newly qualified therapist to embrace the joys and challenges of being in practice.

Continuing professional development is an ongoing theme, emphasising the importance of reflection, supervision and further study. Lots of hints and tips again are provided and the authors reinforce much of what has been encouraged as good practice throughout the graduate's degree study. It is so good to see the emphasis being placed upon the practitioner to take responsibility for maintaining their CPD, not seeing it as a chore but as an opportunity to be embraced throughout their working life.

Models and frames of reference for practice are given a much-needed boost in Chapter 3, whereby the newly qualified therapist is bluntly told that they are just as important in the real world as they were in the academic world. This is so encouraging to see that academic underpinning that contributes to student development of clinical reasoning is being given equal credibility within the practice arena.

The remaining chapters provide excellent advice around the various areas of practice that the newly qualified practitioner may come across in their first post. Alongside this are sections on moving and handling and legislation adaptations – all of which will provide the therapist with invaluable guidance in whichever area they choose to work. Sean's guide to surviving in the acute setting is enjoyable reading, not only for the graduate but also for the student on placement – who often finds the challenge of the acute busy ward environment overwhelming and they struggle to see how the OT process is played out in this environment. Sean's advice is to be welcomed: put the patient at the centre of your care, actively listen to what they have to say, step into their shoes and be genuine and empathetic. The therapeutic use of self is emphasised throughout.

Melanie provides an insightful chapter on being a paediatric occupational therapist and is welcomed, I'm sure, by many graduates who aspire to this role. It is easy to read and broken down into manageable 'chunks', with pointers to further recommended reading. A great guide to this area of practice.

Sara tackles the challenge of guiding the graduate through the complexities of working within mental health. It is good to see the emphasis on teamwork, the occupational process and the importance of reflection. I particularly like the section on the value of group work and how it can be delivered in the community for people with mental health needs. Group work is a great passion of mine and a skill that is essential for all occupational therapists to develop, whatever area of practice they decide to work in. Sara ends with a simple note that as occupational therapists we are here to encourage individuals to identify and set goals, to work collaboratively and to use our creativity in helping individuals on their path to recovery.

Within the chapter on learning disabilities, Ruth's passion shines through; her many years of experience have produced a chapter that is a great guide for anyone contemplating working in this area of practice. Again, there is a strong emphasis on collaborative working – with individuals, their carers and the wider care team. There is recognition that people may have a learning disability but may also experience other issues such as dementia, physical health concerns and mental health needs. The key advice that Ruth provides is to see everyone as an individual.

Two very informative chapters follow, written by the editors of the book, Ruth and Julia. These chapters introduce the graduate to the world of social care, both with children and adults. Clarity is given to the legislation and Acts that underpin this area of practice along with excellent guidance to working in social and community care. Ruth speaks of the social model of disability, hearing the 'voice' of the child, safeguarding and equipment provision. Some excellent reflections are provided. Julia and Dawn present some very practical tips and guides throughout their chapter on adult care and illustrate the positive impact that occupational therapists can have – not just on the individual but also on the family, enabling people to live meaningful and purposeful lives within their homes and community.

Concluding chapters within this essential guide explore in greater detail issues such as manual handling, legislation, governance and data protection, all very important information for the newly qualified graduate.

The pleasure for me in writing this foreword is amplified by the fact that I know many of the writers. Some I have trained, some have provided excellent placement opportunities for my students and all are truly remarkable practising occupational therapists who have a passion for their profession and understand only too well the added value that occupational therapy can bring to individuals, families and the community.

I hope that new graduates to the profession will recognise the passion with which this book has been written and will not only absorb the facts, hints and tips but will also embrace the message that all these writers put forward – that occupational therapy is a wonderful profession and it is a great privilege to have the opportunity to work with people and to make a difference in their lives.

Dr Theresa Baxter
Principal Lecturer in Occupational Therapy
Sheffield Hallam University

Foreword

I had just graduated with my diploma and found myself walking up the drive of the old asylum to the occupational therapy department, which was housed in a couple of leaking wooden huts beneath some conker trees. Approaching this rather dilapidated building I had a growing sense that despite the previous three years study and placement experience, the learning process had really only just begun. Over my first week I discovered that the technical instructors and therapy assistants had many years of experience and regarded the qualified staff as temporary. There was an institutional culture embedded in years of old psychiatric practice. Within that, there was a sense of struggling to develop or at least maintain occupational therapy despite that powerful set of forces, which manifested itself in petty antagonisms between some, though not all, ward staff and the occupational therapy department. There were many things to find out about, toes to step on, mistakes to make, and corners to have knocked off. The background to all these mysteries could be discovered by talking to the man who had the job of changing light bulbs around the old hospital. By virtue of his strange power of taking half an hour to change a bulb, he could slip unobtrusively into many departments and offices, and 'earwig'. One of my new colleagues told me that I had 'to make a plan to leave within eighteen months, or risk becoming as institutionalised as the rest of the staff'.

In the 1990s, many clinicians tended to think of long-term psychiatric care as a backwater. I quickly became very interested in enduring mental health conditions but I had not been prepared for the effects of years of incarceration on people, and found that the challenges were sometimes overwhelming. Colleagues of all disciplines and some of the service users I worked with encouraged me to develop skills, interests and further knowledge. Over time I developed an increasing passion for the fundamental things the profession is striving to achieve, which I would sum up as working for meaningful life opportunities and life quality.

Nonetheless, there was much to enjoy in that first setting, and I moved through the wards, progressing to acting head occupational therapist in a few years. However, along the way, I got things wrong, was over-worked and burned out in ways that are warned of in these pages; but I survived to reflect that this was in large part due to the way that I had approached my new career. I was trying to push ahead too fast, when in fact, there would always be more learning to acquire and ways to work, and always more experience to consolidate. Since then there have been many technological changes, theory and practice developments and innovations in treatment, but many aspects and challenges of occupational therapy work remain very much the same.

In the UK the occupational therapy profession is at a very interesting time. Having expanded rapidly in the post-war period during the first decades of the National Health Service, occupational therapy now has to prove its value as what was once a publically funded service moves increasingly towards the marketplace. New modes of intervention, care pathways, service configurations and partnerships in the organisation of care provision are being put into place. There are lots of new opportunities to navigate, and some of them might require careful consideration, particularly as a newly qualified graduate.

Each chapter of this book provides inside information about what you need to know as you make the transition from student to employee. It is put together by a good range of occupational therapists working in different areas, people with varied life and professional experience whose aim is to tell you like it is. Written conversationally, but based in the wisdom that has been picked up in practice, the text gives sensible, straightforward advice. The writing team have taken into account the dynamics of change affecting healthcare in the UK, including the effects of austerity measures, staff shortages and tight budgets, the shifts in policy and fragmentation of services, the growth of private companies operating alongside the state sector, developments in information systems and approaches to work. The authors can't tell you everything you will need to understand in every situation, but they offer an excellent grounding in what to expect and how to manage – not just your own survival, but to find opportunities.

Many of your worst nightmares can be avoided if you take the advice here: Ruth Parker and Julia Badger talk about the need to clean up your social media profiles – easily overlooked; they also discuss what happens when complaints are made against you – this can be very scary, but good note-keeping, diary-keeping, record-keeping and maintenance of supervision notes will enable you to survive. Sara Brewin describes her experience of the HCPC audit (I was audited twice in the first few years of this measure – it can be a lot of work and might be a very nasty surprise if you haven't prepared). A key tip from Julia Badger and Dawn Simm for anyone working in the community is to park your car facing the direction you intend to exit before the visit, so you can drive away smoothly.

Aside from these valuable insider details from experienced hands, there are important hints at how and what to prioritise, which key policies and documents to have knowledge of in different clinical areas and in a final important section, there is a guide to handling confidential information in the fluid dynamics of digital exchange.

This would have been such a useful book to have had in my first job. It will help you reflect, guide and encourage you and enable you to plan your development. It might enable you to step back from bruising mistakes, but if you do make them, you may be reassured by the advice it gives. Your future success may even depend on it! Health and social care will always be full of challenges and changes, and occupational therapists have to ride with these to be at the forefront of them. As Sean O' Sullivan says, 'jump on board the rollercoaster', and good luck with your occupational therapy career!

Nick Pollard
Senior Lecturer in Occupational Therapy
Sheffield Hallam University

Acknowledgements

Although our names are on the front of this book's cover, it has required input and support from more than just the two of us.

First, we would like to thank our contributors, families (especially Sam and Tony), work colleagues and all at JKP for their patience and support through the process of bringing this project to its release date, and additional thanks to:

Julie Adams, Sara Blackbourn, Tom Brewin, Viv Chamberlain, Liz Cooper, Karen Dowman, Roger Elliott, Laura Fleming, Ann Hearle, Bronwen Jones, Ammelia May, David McKee, Carol McKinder, National Back Exchange, Kate Nicol, Trisha Nutter, Rachel Russell, Paul Sheehan, Garry, Jessica, Laura and Rachael Simm, Nick van der Wayden and Viva Access.

INTRODUCTION

Hello.

Good practice and good manners dictate we introduce ourselves, and explain our role(s) before getting into the activity we have planned with you, an approach you should be aware of from placements!

Julia

After joining the Royal Navy straight from school, my background originates in health, social care and education in a number of roles. After settling in Lincolnshire I originally had a role at a residential support unit for people with autism. From there I moved to teach life skills at Lincoln College, supporting students with physical and learning disabilities to achieve the best they could. This aim underpins my practice to this day. I joined the Children with Disabilities (CWD) team for the first time as a community care officer (occupational therapy assistant), meeting Ruth at my interview! Four years later I successfully applied for and joined the work-based learning occupational therapy degree course affiliated with Sheffield Hallam University. Twenty-eight intensive months later I graduated and started life as an occupational therapist (OT) in adult social care (ASC) working with people over the age of 65, a job I loved. I decided to leave social care after a restructure moved me to a generic role, as I wanted to retain my occupational therapy skills. So in 2012 I rejoined CWD (and Ruth), later leaving to gain experience on a Band 5 rotation in a general hospital. There I had the opportunity to work in orthopaedics, surgery, stroke rehabilitation and general medicine, later promoted to Band 6 prior to returning to adult social care as a senior occupational therapist. In 2016 I sought an opportunity to return to CWD, enabling me to reduce my hours, yet again joining Ruth! Now, as this book nears completion, I am on the move again, gaining new experience in an emerging role working in Lincolnshire's Integrated Equipment Store.

When she approached me with her cunning plan for this book, I thought about my experience interviewing occupational therapists and realised this might be something worth investing time in. As an occupational therapist with a busy workload and an individual with a full life I am aware time is a precious commodity; investing in this book is important for me as it supports your transition to practice, time being something in short supply in the workplace. My suggestion to Ruth that we make this a collaboration with other occupational therapists was because I strongly felt this book would be enriched by the voices of our colleagues from different settings: voices combining to form a complex picture similar to an embroidered image where all the different threads and stitches form the whole.

Ruth

My route to becoming an occupational therapist was the 'traditional' one, A levels and college (St Andrew's School of Occupational Therapy, if you are interested) at 18, graduating three years later. Taking the traditional route further, my applications at this point were for rotational posts, starting life as an occupational therapist in a unit for adults with learning disabilities. I enjoyed this so much I persuaded them to allow me to extend for an extra two months before moving to a 'care of the elderly' in-patient ward. At this point life intervened, and I found myself moving around the country but remaining in roles linked to care for those over 65. Finally we settled in Lincolnshire and I began my working life here initially in intermediate care, moving on to adult social care. In 2005, looking for a change of direction, I moved to the Children with Disabilities Team. If I was looking for a challenge, then I certainly found it. First, I had to scale a cliff-face in terms of knowledge, I was so far out of my comfort zone! Then there are all the changes introduced over the intervening years requiring yet more adjustment. I am one now of two practice supervisors managing a team of ten occupational therapists. Certainly not where I expected to be all those years ago.

Demonstrating that even occupational therapists qualifying back in the 1980s with decades of practice still need to progress, I returned to study in 2007. An MSc in accessibility and inclusive design under my belt, I thought life would settle down but, no, I then embarked on a PhD which, with a fair wind behind me, should be completed around the time this book is published. I mention this to show:

- Occupational therapy offers variety and challenge, sustaining interest and enthusiasm throughout a (hopefully) long career.
- You are not the only one learning and developing – we all are.

Why add to our busy lives by writing this book? This was not part of the plan at all. In a chance conversation with a social work colleague I (Ruth) learned she was writing a book – her second. This intrigued me, so I asked for details. Cutting a long story short, I learned her first book was written to guide newly qualified social workers through their first year post graduation. I can't claim a 'lightbulb' moment, more a slowly spluttering candle, but an idea lodged in my subconscious, and eventually I looked to see if there were books for newly graduating occupational therapists. I found plenty for newly qualified social workers but none for our profession, plenty on specialist occupational therapy clinical areas but none to help with students' transition to practitioner.

I may have been qualified for 30+ years, but this does not mean I am qualified to write this book on my own. I know my limitations. By this point I liked the idea of the challenge, and wanted to see if I could actually move this on.

Taking time to reflect I realised Julia's wide range of experience was exactly what I needed. At this time she was working in adult social care, so once I had persuaded her to join me for coffee and cake I began my campaign to get her on board. Once Julia had considered my proposal she came back with an excellent suggestion, to get others on board. More coffee and cake followed, and we had a plan – a toolkit with chapters written by occupational therapists currently working in each of the areas we wanted to cover. More coffee and cake later (our preferred method for stimulating thought processes) we came up with a list of colleagues we hoped would join us, and wrote our book proposal form. Sending it off to Jessica Kingsley Publishers, we put it to the back of our minds, being very surprised when they contacted us to say they liked the idea! We then began contacting the occupational therapists on our wish list. Not everyone felt able to join us but networking and recommendations saved the day and our edited book project commenced.

Now is the perfect opportunity to introduce our contributors:

Sean

Sean first encountered occupational therapy as a profession in 2007 whilst working for his local authority supporting service users who required assistance with living independently due to long-term conditions, often resulting in a referral to the occupational therapy team. Wanting to find out more about this profession which helped so many people Sean arranged insight days with local occupational therapists in both social care and healthcare. This enabled him to gain insight into the broad spectrum of occupational therapy thanks to some outstanding, enthusiastic occupational therapists who since qualifying Sean had had the pleasure of working with. Sean applied and was accepted on Sheffield Hallam University's practice-based learning programme in 2010, qualifying in 2013. He started life as an occupational therapist as a rotational Band 5 at the local hospital trust gaining experience in the out-patients team in hand therapy, working with patients recovering from upper limb injuries. He also enjoyed a rotation with the community rehab team, having the opportunity to work with a wide range of patients with complex conditions. Following this Sean transferred to trauma and orthopaedics, here he found his occupational therapy niche and has never looked back. Sean is passionate about ensuring occupational therapy in the acute setting has a pivotal role in the patient journey through the healthcare system, with an emphasis on reablement and recovery, and is enthusiastic about service improvement and promoting our profession.

Melanie

Melanie qualified as an occupational therapist in the early 1990s in South Africa and began work with adult physical disability in an acute setting (burns, strokes, arthritis and neurological conditions). After relocating to the UK she worked across different settings (care of the elderly, orthopaedics, mental health for the elderly in the community) before starting her career in paediatrics.

Initially Melanie worked mainly in community settings, homes and schools, with a short spell working in a paediatric acute setting gaining experience of a wide range of disabilities. Melanie then moved to social care: children with disabilities, before moving to independent practice and pursuing further training in sensory integration (SI), recently completing a diploma in SI and considering completion of the MSc within the near future.

Melanie considers herself fortunate to work alongside many very experienced colleagues who have been a great support and who have taught her a tremendous amount. She feels she has learned the most though from children and families she has been privileged to work with. For Melanie, personal reflection on her own performance at work is ongoing, she never stops learning and growing, welcoming change and enjoying challenges.

Sara

Following the completion of a BTEC national diploma in health and social care and HND in care, Sara was successful in gaining a position as a community support worker within a local adult community mental health team. She had some understanding of this role, due to a previous placement, but at this point in her career was unsure as to what career pathway to undertake but really valued the work with patients.

During this time Sara's supervision was carried out by an occupational therapist, and the approach she adopted followed her supervisor's example. It didn't take long for Sara to identify occupational therapy as her chosen career and, with the encouragement of a very knowledgeable occupational therapist (Cathy) and a supportive team coordinator, applied and was accepted, enrolling on the Lincolnshire work-based learning occupational therapy degree course affiliated with Sheffield Hallam University.

On completing her degree Sara began her career as a Band 5 occupational therapist within a local adult community mental health team. Now qualified for six years, during this time Sara's knowledge and experience has grown, and she now works as a Band 6 occupational therapist in an integrated community mental health team. This role, within a supportive and highly skilled team, requires Sara to deliver occupational therapy interventions alongside an occupational therapist and an occupational therapy assistant, act as the carers' lead for the team and act-up as the team's deputy team coordinator.

Sara reflected how a hot chocolate with a friend lead to an unexpected development – adding writing for publication to her repertoire!

Ruth

Ruth was first introduced to occupational therapy at a careers convention held in the college where she was studying for a BSc (Hons) in health studies. This changed the direction of Ruth's studies and career.

Having grown up with a medical condition requiring many years of treatment, Ruth discovered that her hobby had made a positive impact on her health. As soon as she read more about occupational therapy, she realised she had first-hand experience of the importance of occupation in a person's life and wanted a career in occupational therapy. Having made the decision to leave her degree course, Ruth arranged work experience in a local hospital occupational therapy department. During the same year Ruth applied for and was offered a place at the University Hospital of Wales to train as an occupational therapist.

In 1995 Ruth qualified as an occupational therapist. She returned to Cornwall and worked as a basic grade occupational therapist on the rotation for nearly three years. This provided her with a broad range of experience including learning disabilities. For the next five years, Ruth worked in a community mental health team and an assertive outreach team. In 2003, having moved to Lincolnshire, Ruth had an opportunity to join a community learning disabilities team where she remained for the next 11 years. In 2014 Ruth returned to Cornwall to continue working in a community learning disabilities team. Ruth feels incredibly privileged to work with so many amazing people and with such an inspirational team.

Dawn

Dawn qualified as an occupational therapist at the College of Ripon and York St John in 1983. During her time in York she met her husband Garry who was training in the Royal Air Force. Throughout the earlier years of their marriage they moved frequently, mainly up and down the beautiful east coast of England and Scotland, with a period in Hampshire.

Dawn has worked in general and psychiatric hospitals, but following each excursion into health work she returned to her first love – a community occupational therapy role. During a career break to raise her family, Dawn completed an Open University degree course, attaining a BA Hons. Returning to a work environment Dawn spent some time as an activities coordinator in a care home. She also completed care shifts and would recommend this as invaluable experience for anyone involved in hands on moving and handling. A 'return to practice course' completed with the University of Derby provided a theoretical refresher with practical updates at a large general hospital.

Dawn is currently based in a community team with adult care in a market town with a widespread village and rural community. In her spare time she enjoys swimming, cycling, reading and chocolate!

Jo

Jo qualified as an occupational therapist from St Loyes School in Exeter in 1996. Since then, she has worked in a broad range of settings in community and residential services, including time spent in Romanian orphanages. She has developed specific expertise in working with children with complex disabilities in a social care setting.

Throughout her career Jo has had a particular interest in manual handling. She worked as an assessor for a national equipment company for several years, specialising in the assessment and provision of hoists and slings. Jo is an Institute of Occupational Safety and Health (IOSH)-accredited moving and handling trainer and has also worked as an independent occupational therapist.

Currently Jo has a role within the Children with Disabilities Team, enabling her to utilise her extensive knowledge both on supporting children with disabilities and their families, and also promoting and supporting the use of safe moving and handling techniques in her own casework and assisting colleagues with their decision-making in this area of practice.

Kate

Kate is a well-respected occupational therapist, with 30 years of clinical experience, specialising in housing for the last 25 years. She is a director of The OT Service, providing occupational therapy services to case managers and consultancy to companies and individuals on the needs of disabled people and those aged 50 and over. Kate continues to work with individuals, housing associations, insurance companies and individuals to maintain a close link to the grass-root needs of clients and customers, as she passionately believes every client is an expert in their condition; this enables her to keep developing her skills.

Kate has been chair of the Royal College of Occupational Therapists (RCOT) specialist section – Housing and the genHOME project – and represented RCOT in Europe (Council of Occupational Therapists for European Countries – COTEC). She is presently on the team editing the third edition of the *Wheelchair Housing Design Guide.* She also worked with Bristol University on the publication of *Minor Adaptations without Delay*, funded by the Housing Corporation and RCOT and part of the team who developed a Housing MSc pathway with York St John's University.

Kate has presented her work on inclusive design and housing standards nationally and internationally, including Australia, Bosnia, Croatia and Greece, and is also passionate about promoting products and adaptations meeting functional need but also considering aesthetics, as she believes a home should be a place where a client wants to be and not look like a clinical institution.

So what are we trying to achieve with our toolkit? How is this going to assist you as you transition to your new role as a qualified practitioner?

We can't provide you with the 'how' for each and every situation you will encounter. We have painted pictures of occupational therapy in the real world, created by people working in these clinical areas. Not every area – the book would be huge – but those most frequently considered by new graduates. You may have been lucky enough to have experienced these areas as a student, but during placements you are protected in many ways, supported by a placement educator and your university. Placement educators plan your time in their departments considering learning opportunities, adjusting their responsibilities, ensuring you will have the time you need with them. By your final placement you will have become increasingly autonomous in your actions, but still with a high level of support and oversight. Now, following induction, you are expected to take responsibility for your actions and decision-making with reduced support. This is it, the real world.

Not everyone knows where they want to work, which clinical area to choose. We may be able to assist in making this decision as one chapter may stand out from the rest. Alternatively it may serve to confirm an area you don't feel comfortable with at this time (never say never!).

Two contributions do not relate to a specific clinical area but are just as relevant nonetheless: Adaptations and Manual Handling. We strongly suggest you read these as there is relevance to *every* area of occupational therapy. You may not recommend adaptations but understanding the criteria and process will assist you to understand why the ramp/stair lift/level access shower your patient needs isn't provided immediately, or why the sensory/therapy room you believe will promote a child's development cannot be funded by a Disabled Facilities Grant (DFG). Your accurate information sets the scene for the occupational therapists who then assess for, and recommend, adaptations and impacts on their therapeutic relationships.

Advising someone they *should/could* have an adaptation funded may appear to be couched in language indicating this is only a possibility. This is not what is heard or understood, possibly leading to disappointment in the future. This may not just impact on relationships, it may lead to a complaint being submitted, as the patient's expectation has not been met. The occupational therapist has completed their assessment and correctly applied criteria but a complaint was almost inevitable. Please consider how you would feel if your patients *came* with expectations you could never meet. How would you feel about a complaint arising from inaccurate information from a member of your own profession?

Manual handling is not only relevant for those working in 'physical' areas. We all move items, so understanding the impact of poor technique offers you protection, as much as providing sound advice to others protects them. Working in mental health or learning disability settings does not mean all your patients will be ambulant or independent in transfers; keeping your knowledge up to date is time well spent.

Whilst the contributions from practising occupational therapists are useful and interesting to read, transitioning into work is more than joining a team or service. You need to prepare yourself for the ups and downs we all face at some point. The chapter on adapting to working life will assist in managing stress we feel in adapting to a new role and environment and through the challenges presented by the current financial climate.

There are 'boring but essential' parts to everyday life and our profession is no exception. The section on information governance and data protection is designed to set these within practice, not to take you through the detail of the legislation.

Ah, yes, legislation, inescapable in any area. It creates the responsibilities and obligations of our parent organisations, resulting in the commissioning of occupational therapy provision, it protects us and our patients/service users and enables provision of equipment and facilities. Legislation is a thread running through all sections and chapters, but to demonstrate the interconnectivity of key legislation and range across clinical areas they have been combined in a table for easy reference. Here you will also find a summary of the Mental Capacity Act 2005, possibly the legislation with the most impact on our current interactions and practice.

We cannot ignore continuing professional development (CPD). Building knowledge, understanding evidence and growing as individuals not only benefits patients and service users, but also ourselves. Learning and developing keeps us enthusiastic about our role and profession. This in turn presents a positive impression for those we meet; remember this includes those with influence and who commission services!

This is not a book designed to be read from cover to cover in one sitting, nor for all chapters to be read in the order they are presented. This is a toolkit, dip in and out, selecting the parts you need at any given time. Toolkits have preferred options but contain additional items, there 'just in case', often rediscovered in times of need. We hope this book will work for you, mainly for your first steps into the workplace, but there for future reference if required.

1

ADAPTING TO WORKING LIFE

Ruth Parker and Julia Badger

Congratulations! You passed your degree, celebrated, reminisced and stored memories about the wonderful experiences and/or opportunities studying occupational therapy and student life can provide. Your Health and Care Professions Council (HCPC) registration paperwork is complete and 'in the bag' – you have remembered to do this, haven't you?

You've dipped into and read the chapters of this book on areas of practice, and may already have job applications, interviews or a job lined up. Now the realisation of starting your (to be hoped long and fulfilling) professional career as an occupational therapist starts. Such exciting times! Some of you will be 'chomping at the bit' to get going, while others may have reservations and feel they are at a 'crossroads'.

Occupational therapy is a vast, multi-faceted discipline. Opportunities to participate in areas of practice you experienced on placements may assist decisions around which direction to take. Equally, you may want to taste the smorgasbord, moving around core areas of practice or role-emerging opportunities. There is no right or wrong way; it is about personal taste and what works best for you. Whatever your choice, please read on, as the following information may help.

Transition from student to professional life

Housekeeping

While packing up your student home, sorting what to keep, recycle or throw away, take time to complete some housekeeping on your online/social media presence too (Twitter, Facebook, Instagram, etc.). This may mean removing images and postings or simply adjusting your privacy settings. Bear in mind you are making the transition from student to a registered allied health professional (AHP). What is acceptable as student behaviour may be perceived differently or negatively by employers or patients/service users. Media sources have many examples of professionals losing their registration because of 'inappropriate' or 'unprofessional' behaviour outside of the workplace identified through their online presence. This is not to say you need to be a saint from now on (please enjoy life and share with others), just be aware of your profile and professional standards.

Settling in to your new community

You may find you will be relocating away from family and friends, either out of choice (yay – dream job) or necessity (phew – got a job). Look for a house/flat share with other professionals or people in work; preferably one where you can rest at night. You will need to rest after a full day at work; expect to feel tired! Make good use of local knowledge or internet search for activities, interest groups, community amenities and facilities. There will be no 'freshers' week', and there is unlikely to be a large group of people of a similar age, experiencing the same excitement and trepidation, the same common factor. It is hard being alone, not knowing a place or people living there. It is also hard to take the first steps in a new environment, you just have to pick your hard.

> **PLEASE BE BRAVE AND JOIN IN**
> Not only will this help you adjust to your new 'home', reducing feelings of isolation and loneliness, but it also helps you integrate with your community, workplace and help hone your signposting skills.

First day in a new job

Think about how you will travel to your workplace and what you need to get through your working day. We hope you will have learned these basic skills from previous employment and practice placements but just in case you have forgotten:

- If possible, take time to make an informal visit and meet members of the team (you may not have had the opportunity to do this at interview).

- Will you be wearing a uniform? What are the rules about wearing uniform to/from work? Is there a dress code?
- Take something to eat and drink; you may not have time during breaks to purchase sustenance.
- Will you need a work diary? Stationery? Notebook? Some employers provide these items, others do not. Ask!
- Factor in travel time and means of transport. Will you be using public transport, driving, cycling or walking? Do not leave this until the night before or the morning of your first day.
- Seek advice on parking and/or traffic congestion at peak times.
- Contact your new manager or mentor if you are going to be late. First impressions count and, though it cannot always be helped, being late for work on your first day is not a good start.

Integrating into the workplace

In the first few weeks of your new role you should have an induction period. How this period is set will be dependent on the environment or area of practice. For example, in a forensic setting there will be a formal training period (anything up to two weeks) where you will learn safety policies and procedures essential to staff (qualified and non-qualified) working in a secure environment. The majority of workplaces will have a mentor scheme: someone organising your induction period and helping you to settle in. Utilise induction time wisely. Ask questions; there are no 'silly' questions. People in the workplace do not mind being asked questions. *They do mind repeatedly being asked the same question by the same person though.* Write the answers down! Complete all compulsory training while you have the time to do it.

Introduce yourself and get to know names and roles of team members, take up opportunities to 'shadow' and observe how they work. A new job equals new information – a lot of new information. If you have a photographic memory, great! If not, get a notebook and write in the following:

- team members' work contact details (phone/mobile/bleep/email)
- contact details of any other teams or agencies useful to your role
- processes/ways of working – if the process is complicated create a flow diagram or a list, any form enabling you to break it down and understand what you need to do (don't be afraid to ask for assistance if you are struggling with this)
- who's who in the wider team or establishment
- how to find work-related paperwork either on the intranet or in the stationery cupboard
- printer ID number and your IT user name
- password prompt(s)
- your staff number (essential for booking training or speaking to payroll/Human Resources (HR)/Information Technology (IT))
- any questions (and the answers) as they occur.

Obviously this list is not set in stone, use it as guidance and add more relevant information to your work role. The notebook will become your work 'bible', keep it with or near you during the day. The information it holds will be invaluable when you are working on your own.

The National Health Service (NHS) has a preceptorship programme for newly qualified occupational therapists. It provides protected time and support to assimilate theory, and to practise skills learned as a student in real-life situations. Other employers may offer similar schemes, and I urge you to actively engage in this opportunity. This effectively supports your continuing professional development, assists integration into working life, evidences progression and consolidates learning experiences, including working collaboratively with others.

Relationships

It can be challenging at times to get along with everyone in the team. You will work with people from a wide range of cultures, backgrounds, personality types, and values and the difference in ages can be vast, from apprentices just leaving school to people nearing retirement age (and beyond).

Consider for a moment, if everyone was the same, if we all had the same learning style or character? Life would be bland, wouldn't it? Either nothing would get completed or we would all be irritated by each other; it's often the mirror reflection of our own flaws we pick out and dislike in others.

TOP TIP

Find common ground, respect the quality and difference in personality, make an effort to listen to others and reflect on what you have learned. Keep the lines of communication open; no sulking!

Attitudes to work can differ too. There will be members in the team with other priorities outside the work environment (family, informal carers for others, or both). They may not have the same enthusiasm and energy as you or the same career aspirations. Try to find common ground and appreciate them for who they are. One of the best working relationships I experienced was with an occupational therapist who is my polar opposite in personality type. If anonymously paired up on paper, as a team-building exercise, I can imagine sharp intakes of breath, a few chuckles of laughter and some mutterings of 'oh no, it will never work'. But we did; we were the 'dream team' (hand on heart). We accepted and respected each other's skills, openly communicated and had a shared sense of humour. And this is the key to getting on with others: communication, acceptance and respect (with a few laughs).

There will be team-building activities or training opportunities; actively engage in these as they help you to develop professionally and engage with team members. If possible, join in with social activities – you don't have to do everything but the occasional appearance helps. During the working day when workloads and caseloads are pressured and heavy, you may be feeling stressed, or observe a traumatic incident and be upset (yes, this does happen), and it's reassuring to be able to turn to people you work with for support because you know they will understand as they may have 'been there' themselves. Equally team members may turn to you for support. It works both ways.

When you are working in a team, for safety reasons it is vital to let other team members know where you are during the day. Sign in/out of the office, update your electronic calendar if you use one, or update the message board. Find out if your team use a 'buddy' system for when you are on lone visits. Remember to call in and let your 'buddy' know you are safely back at work or home. (If you are the 'buddy', check they are safe if they have not contacted you by the agreed time.) Look after each other.

MANAGING A CASELOAD/WORKLOAD

Caseload = The number of cases (patients/service users) assigned to you in a given time.

Workload = The amount of work required to manage your caseload and successfully meet outcomes. The workload reflects the average time it takes you to do the work for each case and complete other non-casework such as training or secondary duties and projects.

Managing and maintaining caseloads/workloads is not a simple task as there are many challenges. Our working environments are progressively more pressured, with increased demands on services and the complexities of individual cases. It is a balancing act affected by reduced budgets, staff turnover, job freeze or difficulties recruiting qualified workers – all whilst managing restructures, implementing changes in legislation and applying time-intensive best practice.

Manageable caseloads/workloads make a real difference in your ability to engage with patients/service users, deliver quality services and achieve positive outcomes. Some employers will be using strategies to make your caseload/workload manageable, for example caseload weighting (a strategy balancing caseloads, tasks and duties).

There are periods when pressures intensify, attributed to a wide variety of situations:

- increased awareness of a condition or maltreatment
- implementation of new legislation and associated impact on eligibility criteria or service remit
- environmental factors such as changes in the weather (e.g. upsurge in fractures from falls)

- economic issues, for example those on low incomes choosing between 'heat or eat' (increased chest infections, pneumonia, self-neglect, etc.).

You only have to read media reports to understand the difficulties health and social care services face in today's economic climate.

As a worker you need to *make judgements and prioritise your workload.* It is helpful to allow time in the morning to quickly triage your caseload and decide how you will make best use of your available time. You also need to be flexible and not get stressed when interventions run over (as they will do). Do not rush your patient/service user to complete an activity. No clock watching; they will pick up on this. Get to know people on your caseload and allocate time when they are at their best. You will be wasting time trying to complete an assessment when the patient/service user is distracted, such as near a mealtime when they are hungry or if they have visitors waiting. If you are unsure how to prioritise your caseload within your area of practice and/or remit, ask! Team members will have tried and tested strategies which can help.

Essentially workload management is about the *balance* between facetime with your patients/service users and paperwork. Fewer distractions can help but equally so can increased communication with mentors and other team members. Sometimes it can take a fresh pair of eyes (that is you, by the way) to look at systems and processes and identify if they meet practice needs. Are any processes inefficient, is there duplication? Discuss in supervision ways you think processes no longer add value. Offer up ideas.

There have been rapid advances in technology during this millennial age. Are there useful tools or have you used technology in another area of practice which would work well for you and your team? There has been an emphasis in social care for 'smart' working or telework such as use of laptops, tablets, smartphones and so on, where staff use a network to securely access systems and work 'remotely'. In some rural areas this is effective for both service and workers as it reduces travel time. However, it has its challenges, including feelings of isolation and disconnectedness from your team; this way of managing your work is also only as good as the technology used.

When caseloads/workloads are high you will find it challenging to take time out to attend training. New practices are time consuming to learn and implement into your current workload, so make allowances for this. You will know what you need to do to complete your job effectively and efficiently but, in the face of competing pressures, you may be required to make compromises. Please do not be despondent, address these issues in supervision and appraisals. This demonstrates you understand your role and your own strengths and weaknesses within it.

Work–life balance

Experiencing a sense of balance in life is an individual and personal concept. You will have read many theories on this and introduced occupational balance or work–life balance into assessments and outcomes for the people you work with. During the transition from student to working professional it may be difficult to get out of the habit of frequent mid-week socialising with friends. (Hey, even I am encouraging you to get out there, socialise and integrate in the local community.) However, you will find your manager is unsympathetic if you roll into work late every morning, exhausted from the activities of the night before. You are being paid to do your job, and there will be an expectation that you will act professionally, be 'value for money' and provide a good service.

It is equally important, with the stress and intensity of work settings, that you do not get sucked into the culture of over-working, staying late or taking work home to complete paperwork, write reports, catch up on emails and other demands.

TIP

Avoid 'work, eat, sleep, repeat'.

Add further stress from family issues or ill-health which increase demands on your time, and we have a classic recipe for burnout and long-term health issues. You will not be effective at work as your ability to function will be impaired.

Getting the work–life balance right can be tricky at times. Some occupational therapists adapt strategies they have learned from their area of practice, such as time management and compromises, but trying to find solutions to the problem can cause further stress. Sometimes you need to say to yourself 'stop, slow down'. Reclaim your breaks during the day, arrive and leave on time and take all your annual leave. Limit time spent reading and answering emails during the day (so time consuming!). Get moving and have an outlet for letting off steam like going for a walk or swim, or take up a new hobby for during breaks.

If you feel the balance is out of kilter, let your supervisor know how you feel so your workload can be reviewed. If it is not possible to reduce current work, they will know not to add additional casework. Build up your resilience to the pressures of work and home life; regain a sense of balance and wellbeing.

Resilience

Resilience appears to be a 'buzzword' at the moment. Essentially it means having the ability to recover or adjust to change; bounce back in the face of adversity, learn from it and be stronger. It is really important for you as an occupational therapist to be able to do this and not to get burnt out, stressed or worn down. The transition from student to professional life is particularly stressful, you have just got your head around starting in your new role, but you may feel you are expected to be an immediate expert. Think about the challenges you have faced to get to this point in your life so far, and you survived. Now you have more challenges to face; it's the rollercoaster of life.

Reflection is an excellent tool to utilise to increase your resilience. Occupational therapists are so good at this; it is core to our ethos and values. Keep a reflective journal – I still have one and dip into it when I experience periods of self-doubt. Choose your preferred model and apply it to an intervention or interaction you experienced. Unpick the core issues then bind them together again and see how it flows. Review what you have learned. Maybe you found a simple error, an 'oh I forgot to do...' Learn from this. Remember it for the future. It could be you did nothing wrong. You worked within your remit or even above and beyond this. Still unpick it. Was there an agenda you were unaware of at the time? Had 'going above and beyond' created a sense of increased expectation from your patient/service user? Learn from this too.

You will feel tired, and at times vulnerable. These are normal human reactions to the intensity of professional life. As occupational therapists we often see, hear or read about extreme traumas people we work with have experienced. You can sometimes feel the physical symptoms of shock. This is when a support network comes in to its own, and you should talk to your manager as soon as possible.

Most employers have a counselling service. You are not weak, asking for help and support is a strength. Learn from experiences and establish strategies to help you manage and recover. Have a plan. It could be something simple, taking ten minutes out, a short walk to ease the stress, fresh air, a tea break or even booking an appointment with the counsellor. Whatever it takes to get you through until you can engage with your support network.

Recognise these signs in others, offer support and signpost to appropriate agencies. I once witnessed a brilliant nurse, the epitome of resilience, slowly break down over the course of a difficult afternoon. She waved off offers of support from colleagues. I bought her a coffee and a chocolate bar, returned to the ward, directed her to the ward sister's office (said she had a call), told her to sit down with a cuppa. She collapsed into the chair and cried. Nothing was said; it didn't need to be. It was a small token, an act of kindness enabling her to stop, think, readjust and move on. And, yes, before you ask, someone had done exactly the same for me when I was in a similar situation. I learned from it and became stronger, grew more resilient.

Complaints/comments/compliments…or… compliments/comments/complaints?

Feedback is good, something we can learn from, add to our reflective practice. The title above is not a typo, we refer to 'the complaints procedure', but look at your organisation's feedback process. I'd wager it refers to compliments, then comments and *finally* complaints. Most of us focus on negatives, but *take on board positive comments* from patients, service users and colleagues, note these for your log, let your supervisor know.

Comments are just as relevant, they may be 'neutral' but result from someone feeling there was something to say. Reflecting on these can result in changes to practice benefiting you and those you work with.

Now, complaints, these are not the totally negative experience you may expect. Like people, complaints come in many shapes and sizes. Those expressed directly to you require a response, and to be registered in the person's record. We don't mean 'you didn't bring me my cup of tea on time' type complaints by the way. Direct approaches need to be responded to/acknowledged, sometimes requiring an apology.

Remember 'I am sorry...' (even if you don't really feel you are in the wrong) can mollify and placate, supporting effective therapeutic relationships.

Formal complaints are subject to policy and procedure, each organisation having their own process. There may be an online method to register a complaint but a letter or email cannot be disregarded just because 'correct process' has not been followed.

Your first step is advising your manager or supervisor, then registering it appropriately. It is hard to hear someone is unhappy with your approach or work, and you can't help but feel defensive and upset. Reading and reflecting on the content of the complaint with support may highlight it is not all about you (we do tend to internalise things!). It may be the core of an issue is about delays, lack of written information, difficulties in accessing a location, things not entirely within your control. Even if the information is about your actions, remember you do not act in isolation. You will have discussed treatment plans or recommendations with your supervisor, they supported your proposals.

This is where commitment to record keeping is key. Clear, concise and accurate records illustrate actions, intentions and understanding of situations and are evidence as if a complaint is lodged. So, what if it is a 'he said, she said' situation? There are always two sides to every situation, and the person writing the letter or email will feel strongly about the issue. Reviewing records of visits or interventions should indicate the 'how and why' of situations. It may be that a complaint refers to a specific visit, being written some time after the event, your recording (completed in a timely manner) demonstrates your view of what occurred or said. Investigations consider both; records made at the time are not written with a purpose of showing you in a good light or deflecting potential criticism, therefore are viewed as an accurate record in the first instance.

This may seem strange, but complaints can be viewed positively. It may be that you did misread a situation? Reflecting on this is part of personal development. Our team investigates complaints appropriately and remedial actions are taken as needed. But it doesn't end there. Different aspects are considered. It may be that a trend is identified, linking this to other complaints received, and as a team we adjust our practice. This isn't always about the individual.

For example, we have hectic working lives and are not always able to respond to emails immediately. How long is 'too long' before responding? What if the email is about an area which is not your responsibility? What if the case is 'dormant'? Reviewing a complaint we reflected and realised there were differences between team members' views and practices. This was discussed and a consensus reached giving a rule-of-thumb timescale for the team to follow.

Any complaint makes for uncomfortable reading, however experienced or confident you are. Try not to let this become something you review over and over again, unpicking every word and inference. This will lead to stress and affect confidence: work with your supervisor and decide to treat it as a learning opportunity. Take control.

See it, do it, show someone else

Finally, you have adapted to professional life and made the transition from student to a practising occupational therapist. So where do you go from here? I am a great believer in consolidating any learning experience and recommend you do the same. An excellent way to do this is by becoming a practice placement educator (remember how scary they were?). Embrace the opportunity to demonstrate and teach the skills you have learned in your first few years of practice. You will be amazed at how far you have come and developed valuable experience, in your area of practice and in life, on the way. Put this down as a training need in your next supervision or appraisal.

Congratulations again, enjoy working life and especially enjoy being an occupational therapist.

2

CONTINUING PROFESSIONAL DEVELOPMENT

Ruth Parker and Julia Badger

A student graduating now is in a strong position; your learning is based on reflection. Developing the art of reflection is the basis for growth as a practitioner and not something left behind as you leave university and enter the real world. Yes, you will have entered a world where you have much to learn and little time to step back and reflect on anything (let alone keep a record of it); but finding time will help you progress and develop.

There is no need to throw out tools used at university and on placement; entering the workplace is a continuation of work you have already put in, not a completely new start. What has changed is access to learning opportunities. Previously, these have been presented to you, now the onus will be on you to seek out opportunities and to consider your learning needs.

Your Health and Care Professions Council (HCPC) registration requires you to source development opportunities and keep records of these. Audits are completed every two years when a percentage of our profession are asked to submit evidence of their continuing professional development (CPD) activities. Having an up-to-date record will certainly ease stress should you be selected, but will also assist in career development, appraisals and completing future job applications. The HCPC website, the Royal College of Occupational Therapists (RCOT), CPDme and TRAMm Tracker are good resources to help identify areas of CPD an activity contributes to (there are others). Please take time to read the reflection by an experienced occupational therapist who found themselves on the 'back foot' when selected for audit (Chapter 6).

Reading

It is a given, isn't it? Well not really. Dependent on your organisation access to journals may now be limited, not all provide Athens or Shibboleth access. All too often you can find a reference to an article but only view the abstract – so frustrating. It may be there are ways of requesting these but certainly not as quickly as before. British Association of Occupational Therapists (BAOT)/RCOT membership gives access to a number of international journals, so is highly recommended. Dependent on location, and local agreements, you may be able to access higher education establishment libraries – ideal if they have an occupational therapist or other allied health professional school, but worth consideration even if they don't. Your organisation or team may have a library with relevant books and articles, but don't limit yourself to these. Consider new publications which your team may benefit from reading and ask if these can be funded.

At this point, not all your reading should be academic; yes, it is important to keep in touch with new developments in practice but, we would argue, in many (most?) areas of practice, understanding experiences of patients, service users and carers improves your ability to empathise. This may be via books from your library, newspaper or magazine articles. These all add to CPD. Just remember these describe personal reflections and cannot be the basis on which practice is founded.

Writing

Skills you have in writing will now be utilised most often in reports and case notes but this should not be the end of your writing activities. First and foremost there are your reflections. Taking time to record thoughts, feelings, outcomes and experiences will, as mentioned before, support your development and lead to becoming a competent practitioner.

There will be other opportunities to write, some linked to service development where you are asked to review an aspect of practice. It may be possible for you to write for your organisation's publications promoting or explaining your service, an information leaflet...many opportunities are out there.

Remember, everything you read has been written by someone. Many of the contributors for this book have never previously written for publication. Fortunately, they agreed to take the leap into the unknown with us. If we can do this...?

Training and learning opportunities

Lectures and seminars may be a thing of the past, and not all of us are minded to plunge back into academia (though this may well come later), but there will be opportunities to grasp.

Mandatory

These courses are inescapable and essential (but we feel they do not really fulfil the spirit and intention of CPD). Each organisation has mandatory courses which must be completed, some once, some annually or bi-annually. Fire safety courses are very useful but do not alter how you develop as a practitioner. Information governance courses are essential but as a learning tool probably have most impact after you have slipped up...

Informal

Your team members and wider team will have a wide range of skills; during your induction period you should have made the most of this. It shouldn't end there; yes, there will be more emphasis on casework, but still make time to consider if a colleague is carrying out an intervention you have not experienced or are not confident in. Ask if you can observe or if you can shadow them; alternatively ask them to observe you as you introduce new skills to your toolkit. Seek out these chances rather than wait for them to come to you.

Semi-formal

These are opportunities such as at Naidex or the OT Show where there are programmes of seminars or demonstrations you can access.

Formal

Your new area of practice may require completion of specified courses. These are good evidence and warrant recording in your CPD – but don't forget to review and reflect on how this new knowledge has impacted and supported your practice further down the line. Not all formal training will be specific to occupational therapy. There may well be courses with more general scope which will be worthwhile. Options are changing constantly so it is worth the time to do some research to see what is out there. The RCOT and Specialist OT Section conferences and regional study days are excellent, for BAOT members (and we highly recommend membership for the many benefits you receive), there are courses listed in *OT News*.

The next step will be to request funding and study leave. The current financial climate means training budgets may well be limited. Our suggestion is, if you are going to request support for a course or conference, do your homework first. Having a strong argument for why attendance will support practice for you, and for the wider team, may be the difference between a request considered or declined. Remember if you don't ask, you won't get, and if you are turned down one year you may be successful the next.

Social media and online communities

In this connected world it is now possible to access support, information and evidence 24 hours a day. There are numerous forums, blogs and groups out there, a quick scan of Facebook or Twitter will confirm this. Our advice is to take your time. Critically review resources you are considering signing up to; apply the same standards as when reviewing articles. Just because it says occupational therapy in the title or group name doesn't mean to say it is accurate or relevant to your practice. A US- or Australian-based resource will relate to their standards of practice, and may be against local policy. On the other hand a UK site may be out of date, inaccurate or just plain wrong! Be selective and remember not to overwhelm yourself. Just because you followed someone on Twitter or joined a forum does not meant you must remain with them for the rest of your career, it's not a life-long commitment!

Your contribution

These days training has to be a two-way street; if you are supported to gain knowledge or information then you will probably need to disseminate this to colleagues. This may be through a presentation or written summary but remember these in themselves are part of your CPD. This sharing of knowledge does not just link to formal learning. You can pass on relevant knowledge or experience from your time as a student, or since you qualified; supporting colleagues through demonstration of a technique or practice development is just as relevant as feedback from a conference.

The previous section touched on online resources, if you want to join the Twitterati or set up a Facebook group, go for it, but just bear in mind your responsibilities in regard to data protection and your employer's standards. The Data Protection section in this book (Chapter 13) is a starting point.

Supervision and appraisal

Processes and timing of both supervision and appraisal depend on the organisation you have joined. The value of these is dependent on the commitment of both supervisor/supervisee and appraiser/appraisee.

Supervision may be a formal process or more informal, it may be with a senior or with peers and may not even be with an occupational therapist. Supervision has two facets; personal supervision should focus on you as a person and as an occupational therapist, considering how you are working now and how best to support your learning. Casework supervision concentrates on practice, assisting with clinical reasoning and progressing casework. It may seem precious clinical time is taken up by a 'distraction', but if supervision is treated as a core foundation on which practice can be developed you will:

- be supported
- develop your clinical reasoning and decision-making
- ensure your supervisor knows you well enough to work with you on developing your career.

There are different approaches to supervision, some formal, some less so. Both Julia and Ruth use an approach often found in children's services – 'Signs of Safety' (SOS) – which in its simplest form asks three questions: 'What are we worried about?', 'What is working well?' and 'What needs to happen?' Asking yourself these, in connection with your personal supervision, as well as for casework, can be a useful starting point. If you are interested in SOS in more detail, the url is included at the end of this chapter. The point here is not so much to say this is a model of supervision you should adopt but, going into supervision or appraisals, being prepared is beneficial for you and your line manager.

Most organisations have annual appraisals which are reviewed as the year progresses. Like most supervision processes these will have formal structure/paperwork pertinent to the organisation. In most cases the appraisal will have a number of facets. First, to review your progress against targets or aims set the previous year. Often these are measured against goals or standards of the organisation. Following this the appraisal looks to set goals which you will work towards for the following year. These will focus on those which are pertinent to you but may also include team or service goals. In some cases there may be a link to performance-based pay where achievement of goals will determine not only pay increments but possibly a small bonus. Whilst pay levels are important, they should not determine the focus of an appraisal. This should always be about *your* progression and development using the core principles of your organisation as the setting these are placed within.

If you already have a clear career path and end goal, identifying learning opportunities and goals can be relatively easy, enabling you to consider what or where you want to be not only in 12 months, but beyond this as well. It might be you have not yet settled in an area of occupational therapy you feel you want to progress in, perhaps in a rotational post. Taking time to reflect on which opportunities are open to you in your current role is important, but so too are considerations of transferable skills. Taking opportunities, in either of these situations, to sit with a more experienced colleague to review, reflect and to plan is invaluable. The outcome of an appraisal meeting should be a clear strategy for the next 12 months, reinforced by goals which are SMART (Specific, Measurable, Achievable, Realistic and Timed), with activities and support identified to assist you in achieving your goals. Once an appraisal is written, don't just file it away with your CPD log and drag it out for scheduled reviews. Consider it every time you add to your log, revise it if you identify new learning opportunities (with your supervisor's agreement) and keep it as a plan which will work for you.

RCOT career development framework

Having a structure or career plan will assist with focusing your CPD and support discussions with supervisors. The RCOT has published a framework (also available to non-members) which supports you in reviewing your progress so far and identifying areas for development across four areas (pillars; Figure 2.1):

- professional practice
- facilitation of learning
- leadership
- evidence, research and development.

Professional Practice	Maintain occupation at the centre of practice. Deliver safe, effective, person-centred and ethical practice. Use professional judgement, reasoning and decision-making.
Facilitation of Learning	Teach, mentor, supervise and/or assess others. Facilitate placement learning. Create and evaluate learning environments, tools and materials.
Leadership	Identify, monitor and enhance own knowledge and skills. Guide, direct and/or facilitate team work. Design, implement and manage professional and/or organisational change.
Evidence, Research and Development	Influence broader socio-economic and political agendas. Create, use and/or translate evidence to inform practice. Design, implement, evaluate and disseminate research.

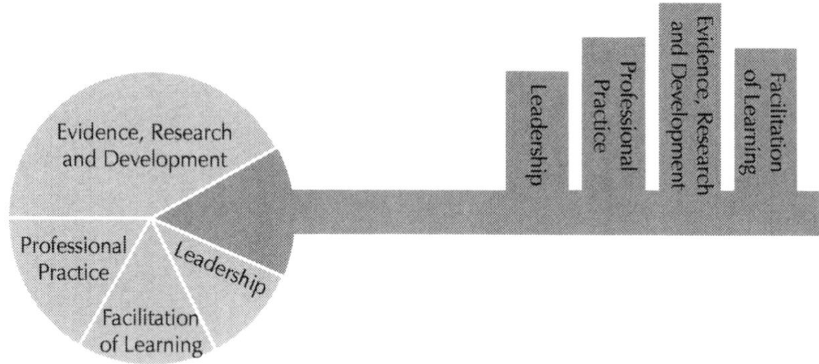

Figure 2.1 The career framework pillars of practice
Source: Royal College of Occupational Therapists (2017) *The Career Development Framework: Guiding Principles for Occupational Therapy.* London: RCOT. Accessed on 13/12/2017 at www.rcot.co.uk/practice-resources/learning-zone/career-development-framework

These are then mapped across nine levels relating to your understanding, knowledge and expertise, the framework document containing detailed explanation of each level. It is likely this new (at time of publication) resource will be adopted by many organisations as the method of planning and supporting career development, therefore having an understanding of the framework is needed and using it to guide your CPD highly recommended.

Part of the purpose of this book is to prepare you for the 'real world'. You may find colleagues don't take this approach, considering appraisal an annual 'chore' and you an 'enthusiastic newbie who will soon realise the error of their ways'. Treat this as a challenge! Not to change their opinions, but to make the system work for you and for your development as an occupational therapist.

To summarise, CPD continues throughout your professional life. It is a foundation supporting practice. To meet our HCPC obligations OTs are required to demonstrate a variety of learning opportunities have been utilised: formal, informal, self-directed, independent and shared. This variety should ensure you remain enthused about your profession, and in the future able to support less experienced colleagues with relevant and informative advice, just as others will have supported you.

USEFUL WEBSITES

Career Development Framework: www.rcot.co.uk/practice-resources/learning-zone/career-development-framework

CPDme: www.cpdme.com

HCPC: www.hcpc-uk.co.uk

Royal College of Occupational Therapists: www.rcot.co.uk

Signs of Safety: www.signsofsafety.net

TRAMm Tracker: www.trammcpd.com

3

MODELS AND FRAMES OF REFERENCE IN THE REAL WORLD

Ruth Parker and Julia Badger

All through your studies models and frames of reference (FoR) are constants – but you are qualified now, they are in your past, you will now be working as an occupational therapist. Actually, no, what happens is they are just as important but less overt. They remain the basis on which we form our practice, our rock or foundation. They are the tools to assist us with our focus on occupation.

Some teams adopt a particular model or FoR throughout their practice, making life 'easy' in your approach to interventions and record keeping. They also provide a common vocabulary to converse in, supporting communication between team members.

Frames of reference then enable you to consider how you will address an individual's identified needs. These are effectively the options available to you within your skill set which you will then use to create your treatment plan.

Now you are expecting us to list and explain each of the key models – wrong. Specific models and FoRs are covered in some chapters relating to areas of practice but here we want to discuss how you manage and relate to models and FoRs whilst adrift in a team who may leave you to make your own mind up.

Personal choice

First – you don't have to pick one and stick with it. Our team have adopted the Person–Environment–Occupation–Performance (PEOP) model to underpin our practice, but this doesn't prevent us considering a situation through the lens of the Model of Human Occupation (MOHO) or Kawa River models.

If you have had a placement with teams who have a strong relationship with a particular model then you may find you have settled comfortably with that. It may be in job hunting you will focus on those job adverts highlighting 'your' model.

But life isn't as simple as that. These days getting a job may mean joining a rotational post, choosing a post based on location or simply because you have been successful at interview (those student loans and everyday expenses need to be funded!).

How do you cope? If a team has a strong affiliation to a particular model you don't feel the same way about, be open minded. If you find the PEOP model 'speaks' to you most, but you are in a mental health setting which is MOHO through and through, take time to look for overlaps. Reflection is such a useful tool to help you find your way through this, but on a practical point there is no point in swimming against the tide and trying to impose 'your' model – flexibility is vital.

Teams without a defined model may seem the easy option. You can join them, become established in practice and no one will ever challenge you to explain *how and why* you came to your treatment plan – well, until you take on your first student. Then any student worth their salt should be challenging you to explain, as this is how they will (and you did) understand the link between theoretical models, FoR and practice.

It is like trying on shoes. You have an occasion to attend, an outfit to wear, but you need to find shoes which fit the occasion, suit the outfit, but most important will be comfortable to wear.

Discussions with others

So, you have your model and are comfortably working within it. Sometimes with other members of the multi-disciplinary team (MDT) discussing your approach assists their understanding of your treatment plan or proposals. But what about with patients, service users and carers?

In mental health an in-patient unit may operate within the framework of a model, requiring patients to cooperate within its parameters for interventions to be effective. This will require discussion with patients to ensure they understand the ethos to optimise impact of their interventions. It may also require discussions with family members or carers; their support and understanding are as important as the patients' in achieving the desired outcome.

The example above gives clarity where a model is adopted but we circle back to those less-defined areas. Should you be explaining your approach in detail?

Yes and no. We know this book is supposed to assist with answers but, using the toolkit analogy, this is a situation where a specific size of spanner, an adjustable one, pliers or mole grips will all tighten the nut. Explaining your approach may assist a patient or service user – or may confuse the issue. Describing the Motor Learning Model as a way of teaching handwriting to a parent may be helpful for their understanding of how to support their child. Using the Kawa River Model with an elderly patient to support discharge planning may help you but, in many cases, they will be looking at you askance! It is a case of considering each situation and acting as you see fit.

Frames of reference – where do these fit? (Analogy alert!) We are heading for the kitchen now – the spice rack to be precise. You have planned a meal – Chinese, Italian, Indian, Thai…the choice is yours, but this is the model you are adopting. To create your dish (treatment plan) you will select the appropriate spices (FoR). You will become an 'inventive chef' as you grow as an occupational therapist. At first you will have a limited repertoire, maybe relying on ready-made spice mixes. As you increase in knowledge, experience and confidence your ability to select the most appropriate mix of FoR will develop.

This leads on to clinical reasoning. Did you ever wonder what was going on in the brains of the occupational therapists you met on placement? How did they come to the 'snap' decisions they made? How did they decide assessing for a bath board and seat could be missed out and their first step is to try a bath lift? This is the wonderful thing called experience. At first you will need to take every step of the assessment process, working through the activity analysis in detail. Yes, this is slower, but this is where you build up all those snippets of information and experiences essential to your development. In time you too will be able to take these 'short cuts'.

This has dealt with the thinking part of things but the records need to reflect this too. Your clinical reasoning needs to be written down so your actions can be understood. The box shows a simple example.

PLANNED INTERVENTION: ASSESSMENT WITH BATH LIFT

Mrs X has insufficient postural control to use a bath board and seat to access the bath, requiring a backrest for trunk support. Her lack of upper body strength means she would not be able to support herself during transfers on/off a bath seat. A bath lift offers the support required via backrest and will raise/lower her from the base of the bath.

Simply noting you opted to assess with a bath lift is not an accurate reflection of your clinical reasoning, therefore noting why you have discounted other options gives a full picture.

Some models such as PEOP provide a framework for writing up assessments and interventions. These guide your thought processes and ensure all essential information gathered is recorded. Assessment recording may be 'formal' with sections dedicated to specific areas, for example spirituality, environment, occupations...or could be task focused, requiring you to consider the FoR for each task.

As identified in the opening paragraph of this section, models and FoRs are a constant in an occupational therapist's working life, supporting both practice and the presentation of our interventions. Neglecting this essential aspect of practice is an error you may regret in the face of a challenge or questioning of your decision-making processes. Embedding them into your practice is well worth a little bit of time and effort.

4

THE ACUTE HOSPITAL SETTING

Sean O'Sullivan

Introduction

Welcome to the acute hospital setting, the rollercoaster ride new graduate occupational therapists can experience as a place to cut their teeth, learn their trade and cut away those apron strings. As an occupational therapist starting at Band 5 level you will be spending a set period of time working across different wards with a variety of specialties, otherwise known as being 'on rotation'. You will have the opportunity to work on medical wards, surgical, trauma and orthopaedics, oncology, cardiology, stroke and neurology, paediatrics and perhaps more, depending on the hospital where you are employed. The length of time spent in each area will of course be different, depending on where you will be working, but typically you can expect to spend six months in any clinical area. This will give you plenty of opportunities to shake off the student comfort blanket and stretch your wings, because you will be working with patients with a variety of health problems impacting in one way or another on how they do things, making them unique occupational beings.

Have I sold it to you yet? Are you queuing up to join us on the rollercoaster? Well, before you do, just take a step back, think again and consider whether this is really for you. Look how fast the ride is going, look at all the loops and frightening turns you will be going through at breakneck speed, without ability to control the acceleration, or number of turns and loops you will go through. Just look at the size of the queue waiting to get on. What happens if the ride breaks down and you can't get off? What happens if it won't stop and just keeps going round and round?! There is an awful lot I haven't mentioned yet. Most importantly you need to understand the context of the environment you are about to jump head-first into as a highly enthusiastic, newly released graduate occupational therapist, bursting with ideas and preconceptions of what it means to be an autonomous practitioner in the acute sector.

First of all, it will be highly likely that you will be working in a National Health Service (NHS) hospital. If you have little interest or haven't been paying attention to the problems the NHS faces in terms of limited budgets and resources to deliver the very best treatment and care for our patients (who by the way are living longer with more complex health and social problems), then read no further; working with patients in the acute hospital sector isn't for you.

I have to be honest, if you want to be the occupational therapist you want to be, or are capable of becoming, you need to know you will be facing an uphill struggle all the time. You won't have all the resources you need; you will have a demanding caseload. You will be constantly harassed by your colleagues, team leads, heads of service, nurses, doctors, consultants, bed managers, complex case managers, discharge coordinators and a seemingly endless number of people above this level who all generally want to know the same thing. Is this patient medically fit for discharge? When can this patient be discharged from hospital? Guess who they all come to for the answer – yes, you!

Context and challenges

Right, down to business. The NHS as we know it really is under a tremendous amount of strain. The Kings Fund (www.kingsfund.org.uk) is a fantastic place to start your research into the many challenges we face, what we don't do so well at, where we excel and where possible solutions to our problems may be. To gain an understanding of the direction we are heading with the delivering of health and social care nationally, look also at the *Five Year Forward View* (NHS England 2014). Locally you should be able to locate information on the transformation agenda, which is set to shape our future services. The key messages in all of these policy drivers are about delivering first class patient care (patients are at the centre of everything we do) in the most appropriate environment, to get the best outcome. If there is a genuine need to be in hospital, you obviously need to be there. If your needs can be treated or managed away from this environment, then you don't require a bed in an acute hospital setting, period. Health and social care will look to move patients to the most appropriate place at the earliest opportunity. The hope is this is back to their home, where generally people recover faster and have a better quality of life.

Significant problems often cause delays and disruptions to the flow of patients moving through the acute hospital sector. There are huge pressures on accident and emergency (A&E) departments to see patients as per government standards. There are also huge pressures on ensuring there are enough beds to meet demands for patients requiring hospital admission. These pressures continue in the community setting, where health and social care need to ensure there is sufficient care in the community to support patients on discharge. If any one of these areas struggle, which they invariably do, the system becomes blocked.

So where do we as occupational therapists fit into this? This will depend on the area where you work but essentially you could be involved with all aspects of the patient journey through the acute hospital setting. Therefore it is important to understand the role of the occupational therapist in this setting. It is not just about washing and dressing assessments, providing equipment to assist with daily living or establishing the level of care someone may need when they leave hospital – all of which we are involved in but only as part of a much wider scope of practice. You will be adding zero value to the patient experience or to their discharge from hospital if you simply report that a patient recovering from a fractured hip cannot wash their lower half. Equally applicable is reporting that a patient with dementia, who normally manages just fine within their own routine at home, cannot make a cup of tea in the occupational therapy kitchen. You will be expected to practise at a deeper level than this. Let's explore our role further.

Scope of practice

In my hospital trust I work across the surgical wards, mainly trauma and orthopaedic, which have become my specialty. I will explain the role of the occupational therapist in this context because you are highly likely to have a rotation in in this area. A high percentage of patients who are admitted to hospital are 80+, often following a fall associated with frailty. Consequently, a high percentage of these patients end up with a fractured neck of femur. You will, wherever you are on rotation, come across patients who tick one, if not all of these boxes. For further reading on this I suggest the National Audit Office (2016) report *Discharging Older Patients from Hospital.* The number of people who fall sustaining a fractured neck of femur has been identified as a major public health issue due to the ever-increasing ageing population. Approximately 65,000 hip fractures occur each year. Of these, about 10 per cent of people die within one month, and one-third within 12 months (National Institute for Health and Care Excellence (NICE) 2017a). Up to 20 per cent of this population require long-term care post fracture, and a further 30 per cent do not return to their pre-fracture functioning. Hip fracture accounts for 87 per cent of total fragility fractures (Age UK 2017; NICE 2017b). Therefore working in trauma and orthopaedics is challenging and represents a broad scope of practice for occupational therapists.

The main aim of occupational therapy-focused rehabilitation in trauma and orthopaedics is similar to the concept of recovery in many mental health settings. It is about recovering ordinary lives and enabling patients to progress as best they can, so they can live as they choose, for as long as they are able. Putting recovery into action means focusing care on supporting and building the resilience of our patients, not just on treating or managing their symptoms. The guiding principle is hope – the belief it is possible for someone to regain a meaningful life, despite serious injury.

This is a really important message. Ultimately, we can never say to a patient 'Don't worry, you will never fall again.' We can never tell a patient they will manage at home risk free – it is not realistic, it's not a true reflection on life; we don't live in utopia. What is realistic is supporting patients to re-establish their abilities to 'self-care' as best they can, to encourage positive as opposed to detrimental risk taking, thereby reducing the need to rely on others for support. The occupational therapist is typically involved the whole way through a patient's journey.

Triage and referral

In my workplace we have a 'blanket' referral system, by which I mean there isn't an expectation on the ward for teams to 'refer' a patient to occupational therapy. We see everyone, most of our patients will have sustained a fracture because of a fall, and there are national standards and local trust standards we need to adhere to. However, if I see every patient who has fallen and sustained a fracture, this may mean I am involved with up to 56 patients across two wards; this isn't sustainable. As I explain the role of the occupational therapist in more detail you will understand why.

Leaving patients with fractured neck of femur aside, as a Band 5 occupational therapist you will need to develop skills in the triage of patients to help you determine whether you, as an autonomous practitioner, can add any value or proactively contribute to a particular patient's care, recovery and discharge from hospital. The key to this is your ability to gather all relevant information you require to inform your decision. You can do this through a variety of methods such as looking at why they were admitted, how they sustained the injury, seeing if they had recent admissions, entries from the ambulance crew, records at A&E. Also, initial information gathering from the patient, contacting family and friends (with patients' permission) and, if appropriate, speaking to the care home manager. Remember at this stage you are still gathering information, you haven't decided to proceed to assessment yet, you are considering whether it is essentially worth your time and, most importantly, the patient's time, getting involved or not. If you do not feel you can make a positive contribution then there is no obligation to get involved, as long as you can give clear clinical reasoning for not doing so. This aspect can be particularly difficult for a Band 5 to accept. It can also be incredibly challenging to justify why you won't get involved to the multi-disciplinary team, to families and even to the patient. But if you are to manage a demanding caseload this is essential.

If you lack the confidence to challenge appropriately there is a risk your role as an occupational therapist will then be defined by others and before you know it you are shaped and moulded into the occupational therapist others want you to be. We are all autonomous practitioners, if you go down this line, I promise you, you will not develop further in the acute hospital setting. Also, what does this say about the unique value of occupational therapy in this setting? Are you just duplicating what other professionals should be doing? Invariably, as with any work setting, people will take advantage of this!

Assessment

Having considered all the information to hand, after discussions with the patient, family and health and social care professionals involved, you decide you can justify having this patient on your caseload and there is potential for occupational therapy to have a positive impact. You then proceed to assessment.

Establishing a therapeutic relationship with your patient is key to enabling patients to be proactive with their rehabilitation and recovery, so it is important to hit the ground running. This involves the therapeutic use of self, building rapport, trust, respect, sincerity and empathy with the patient.

Every patient is different. The approach you took with patient A will not necessarily work with patient B, and you will have to adapt and modify your approach in order to complete a comprehensive holistic assessment. You also must remember the context of what the patient is going through at a moment in time. Most patients we see in trauma have been admitted due to a 'traumatic event', they have had the experience of being admitted for major surgery and are now on an acute trauma ward. Here they may be sharing a bay with five other patients, in close proximity to each other, with only a curtain to give some semblance of privacy. The ward is noisy, incredibly busy, they have a catheter in situ and their hip hurts like hell. A patient is highly unlikely to engage in a 'question and answer' session about how they would normally wash and dress themselves, or whether they make their own meals at home at this time. These questions are not relevant, not appropriate. What is important is empathy, showing you understand what they are going through and reassuring them you are on their side.

I am also a practice placement educator and one of the first things I ask students to do is just to sit with patients and actively listen to what they have to say. Forget the medical jargon, forget the pressures of being on placement, just sit and listen. It is only by doing this that you develop an understanding that the patient is the real agent of change. As occupational therapists we guide, encourage, facilitate, enable but, ultimately, it is up to the patient whether they want to get out of bed or not. Your job is to flick the switch, push the right buttons and your holistic assessment will inform your intervention plan, enabling this to happen.

Simple gestures such finding the patient's spectacles for them so they can actually see who they are talking to, filling up their empty cup as the water jug was out of reach, act as foundations establishing an effective therapeutic relationship. You need the patient to actively engage. If they can tolerate it, sit them up in bed. Consider how vulnerable you would feel if someone was looming over you as you lie in bed, asking questions about how you live your life.

First impressions are important but exactly how do you explain to them you want to start an occupational therapy assessment so you can figure out how to enable them to achieve health, wellbeing and life satisfaction through participation in occupation?!

First, remember what the patient has been through. You're probably the tenth person who has spoken to them at their bedside today, they're tired, in pain, fed up of people asking the same questions over and over again. There is a time and a place to proudly proclaim the language of occupational therapy in all its splendour and glory, but at this stage I often go for:

> Hi, I'm Sean, I'm an occupational therapist and I'm involved with your rehab and recovery but I'll go into that a bit more later... (a quick precursory glance at the injury site). Oooof! That looks nasty, what happened to you?!

Of course, every patient is different, it comes down to your own clinical judgement and life experience on whether to take a more formal approach or not. At the triage stage you should have gleaned enough information to inform which approach you will select. Generally, I find the above approach very effective. I've introduced myself without bombarding the patient with information, I've empathised with the patient and I genuinely want to know what happened from the patient's perspective. How they feel their injury/illness will impact on their life is absolutely essential and should directly inform your assessment, intervention plan and goal setting.

As a Band 5 on rotation it will be important to know the kinds of injuries, illnesses and medical conditions relevant to the clinical area. What is more important is helping the patient to identify and deal with the impact of the illness/injury. There are plenty of medical professionals involved with your patient purely looking at them from a medical perspective. Your job as an occupational therapist is a balance between having a good understanding of the medical model and a more thorough understanding of how the patient's current situation impacts on their ability to engage in occupations mattering to them.

Let the patient talk with minimal interruptions at this point, and remember they are expert in how they live their life.

Use all your occupational therapy knowledge and skills to develop a holistic understanding of the person's situation. A patient who has sustained a wrist fracture, for example, now in a cast, unable to actively use their dominant hand, may be 'medically' fit to be discharged from hospital from an orthopaedic point of view. But it's your job as an occupational therapist to work with them to identify the barriers and enablers to recovery – and it isn't all about the ability to manage personal care. Very often it is dealing with situations such as 'If I can't use my wrist I can't push my husband's wheelchair. If I can't push the wheelchair I can't get him to day care, I'm his carer, I need that break!', or 'I've just finished six weeks of radiotherapy, I'm absolutely wiped out, which is why I think I fell in the first place.' Frequently it's 'I tried to get out of bed and slipped off the edge again' and 'I couldn't manage without using my kitchen trolley at home, but they tell me I can't use this wrist.' Your assessment shouldn't only be about identifying reduced functional ability to use the affected wrist. It's about what this means to the person, how this will change their situation and how they will need to adapt and compensate to overcome the barriers. You will be picking up on any cognitive deficits, behavioural aspects, their level of insight in terms of risk, ongoing mental and physical health problems impacting on recovery. Also consider how the patient would normally overcome these barriers, their social network, family dynamics and home environment. Your occupational therapy brain will be busy processing this information to formulate an intervention plan based on what the patient wants to achieve, and requires for a successful discharge from hospital.

Goal setting

In the acute setting it can be very difficult to get patients to identify clear occupational therapy goals. If only I had a penny for every time a patient said to me 'to get walking'! Our physiotherapy colleagues come into their own with this type of goal, and you will generally find patients initially more receptive to physio goals. This is fine because it's OK to conduct joint assessments with physios on aspects such as transfers, mobility, balance, gait, strength and range of movement in the initial stages of rehabilitation. This informs the patient and the occupational therapist in setting a nice meaty occupational therapist-focused SMART (Specific, Measurable, Achievable, Realistic and Timed) goal. If your patient wants 'to get walking', it's always a means to an end. A good way of breaking this down is to go through their daily routine with them. Use your activity analysis skills to break down specific tasks they hope to be able to return to when they get home. The 'get walking' evolves into 'to get to the bathroom and manage my personal care independently' or 'so I can return home and continue caring for my wife who has dementia'. On one level it's good to see a patient mobilising a few steps with a walking frame, but is this going to work for them at home? Will the prescribed walking frame be conducive to the patient's needs in their home environment? How can he help his wife cook dinner if he is too reliant on the walking frame?

Intervention plan

At this point you have established a therapeutic relationship with the patient, conducted a comprehensive initial assessment, helped the patient identify goals to work towards and now you need an intervention plan. Patients often become passive recipients of care in hospital, and you will be astounded at how quickly a normally active, independent person becomes bed bound. This 'pyjama paralysis' is very difficult to shake off once it sets in. It is also highly infectious, and you will notice other patients in close proximity exhibiting similar behaviours. In no time at all you have a full bay of patients on your caseload, 11am, still in bed, lying flat, eyes closed, bed sheets pulled up to their chins in a kind of dreamy-like state. Engaging the patient as an active participant with their rehabilitation, recovery and discharge planning becomes similar to pushing an elephant up a flight of stairs.

Enabling patients to be active participants at the earliest possible stage is essential. Intervention plans empowering patients and giving ownership are often more effective than plans focusing on baseline assessments, such as 'washing and dressing assessment' or 'kitchen assessment'. These do have a place in the occupational therapy toolbox, but it comes down to your own clinical reasoning on how and when to use them. Conducting a washing and dressing assessment two days after major surgery will be a waste of your clinical time and have little benefit for the patient. Building good relationships with healthcare support workers on the ward who work with patients every day and can reinforce the goals you have set with the patients is key. Setting a daily goal for a patient to work towards, such as managing an achievable personal care task, followed by getting dressed into day clothes every morning, is more effective, maintaining participation and ownership of their rehabilitation and recovery. You can review this with the patient at any time and then set further daily goals using a graded approach.

Ultimately the intervention plan will be centred around the goals you and the patient want to achieve. However, in the acute setting there are key areas to address. Whether the patient lives at home, is going to stay with relatives on discharge or lives in a care home, you will be assessing if this environment is conducive to the patient's needs. This includes recommendations and/or provision of equipment, recommending alterations to the property, minimising the risk of falls and working with patients to establish a support network of friends, family and/or formal carers to help facilitate their recovery. This is essentially discharge planning and should run parallel with a patient's progress for the best possible outcome.

Keep in mind the following:

- Overloading a patient with equipment to assist with activities of daily living (ADL) is not the solution.
- Never assume friends and relatives will support on discharge.
- What's a clear falls risk to you may not be considered a risk by the patient at all.
- Something unexpected *will* crop up at some point which has the potential to jeopardise your whole plan unless it is resolved as quickly as possible!

With the patient's consent, it is vital to meet with relatives/carers at the earliest opportunity, start establishing a rapport and break down any barriers. You will meet some fantastic patients where family and friends rally round and everything goes seamlessly but it's not always like this, be prepared to have some difficult conversations; during the patient's admission, this means dispelling any myths around what happens on discharge and also managing expectations.

Positive risk taking

As I have already outlined there is huge pressure on hospitals to discharge patients who are medically fit at the earliest opportunity. At some point you will arrive at the conclusion you have taken your patient as far as you can. They have engaged with the intervention plan, worked towards achieving their goals, their recovery can be managed away from the acute hospital setting.

Now you need to be brave enough to let them go despite the risks associated with this! We always emphasise with patients and their families we aim for 'home first' and have a 'reablement' approach. Re-establishing a familiar daily routine back at home, with the appropriate level of support in place, is by far the best outcome. However, not everyone will necessarily agree with you on this. Patients and families are understandably very apprehensive at this stage. They want reassurances all will be well when they return home, they won't fall again, they will get back to doing things they enjoy at home. You simply cannot offer these assurances, life itself is inherently risky. Nothing is 'risk free' and we are all capable of making unwise decisions leading to illness or injury. All we can do is acknowledge these facts of life and try to manage the risks as best as we can. This is the key message you will have to get across to patients and families.

It will become apparent during your transition period as a newly qualified occupational therapist in this setting that having a caseload of vulnerable patients may lead to the overwhelming fear you might 'get it wrong' somewhere along the line. Your caseload will include patients with unrealistic expectations about their recovery and with a limited insight into the risks associated with some of their decision-making. You will have to deal with families/friends/carers who quite understandably want to protect their loved ones and have very different views about what's in the best interests of the patient. As a Band 5 you should get the appropriate level of supervision from senior occupational therapists, who will support you with clinical reasoning and decision-making, but they won't solve all your problems for you. You cannot 'pass the buck' when it comes to managing risk, especially if you are the one directly involved with the patient and their family.

There are other discharge pathways such as short-term and/or rehabilitation placements before returning home, and patients and families will inquire about these. In some cases these are appropriate pathways to consider, and often seen as the safest solution. It essentially comes down to whether or not you feel confident you have done everything you can in your capacity to manage risks associated with the patient returning home. Are you confident in your clinical reasoning, because of the benefits, are these risks worth taking? On the one hand, if a patient requires further time and education to gain confidence to use their walking frame safely, then a placement setting may be more appropriate. On the other hand, no amount of plodding away with a walking frame for six weeks will emulate their independent daily routine at home – the environments are different. In all likelihood the patient will be no better off, it's wasted their time and raised unrealistic expectations. Also, the placement could have gone to someone who really needed it in the first place.

You will have to acknowledge, despite all your hard work with the patient, all those compensatory techniques, falls risk awareness advice, efforts you have put into improving home layout, equipment provision assisting with ADL, liaising with agencies (such as adult social care) ensuring the right care package is in place, may be disregarded. As long as the patient has the mental capacity to make informed decisions about how they live their life, they are perfectly entitled to ignore all of it, and end up falling again. Expect to have some very frank conversations with your patients. The onus is now on them to take responsibility for their own health and wellbeing and this is entirely out of your control.

Conclusion

Despite the challenges, the NHS is a truly wonderful place to work, offering plenty of opportunities to continue your professional development. There is a real sense of 'we're all in this together', including our patients with whom we have the privilege to work.

I have provided a snapshot of the scope of our role in the acute hospital setting. Trauma and orthopaedics have been explored in more detail to provide you with insight into how we deliver occupational therapy in this setting.

I hope I have informed you about the challenges the NHS faces on a daily basis and signposted you to relevant reading for further insight. These are challenging times for our profession, we are under an increasing amount of pressure to demonstrate the value of occupational therapy in the acute hospital setting. I hope I have got the message across that if our role is merely about provision of equipment, then we are not practising as occupational therapists. You haven't spent three years at university to provide raised toilet seats and perching stools only. Patients are more likely to be concerned about issues related to meaning, values and purpose than worrying about if they can wash their backs independently or make a cup of tea in the occupational therapy kitchen. Your focus should be addressing the barriers and enablers to recovery on the former, not the latter. A multi-disciplinary approach is needed to support patients through their hospital journey, but you must ensure your role remains distinctive. What we do in practice must be occupationally focused and the only way you can do this is to articulate our professional philosophy.

Are you up for the challenge? If so, jump on board the rollercoaster!

5

PAEDIATRIC OCCUPATIONAL THERAPY

Melanie Elliott

Welcome to the field of paediatrics, a diverse and exciting area of practice with many learning and specialisation opportunities.

Roles will vary depending on what your service is commissioned to provide. You may find yourself working in hospitals/acute settings, for example neo-natal intensive care, burns, hand therapy, with neuromuscular conditions, head injuries, juvenile chronic arthritis or with acutely/terminally ill children.

Alternatively, you could be community based, in wheelchair services, social care, mental health services, schools and homes, providing therapy, assessment, intervention, support, advice and training.

Opportunities in private practice are increasing, providing services directly to families though commissioned on behalf of families by case-management companies, schools, colleges or residential placements.

However, the ethos and guiding principles are common to all paediatric occupational therapists. We aim to support development and skill acquisition, prevent deformity and promote access to opportunities, thus maximising a child/young person's potential.

Occupational therapists' knowledge and training enables them to address:

- sensory processing
- motor skills (fine and gross)
- posture and positioning
- manual handling
- perceptual–motor skills (most frequently handwriting)

- feeding and independence skills
- attention and focus
- social skills and behaviour
- task analysis
- environmental and task adaptation including assistive technology.

Examples of activities and interventions to achieve goals you identify include:

- developing physical skills for independent personal care
- participation in social activities or accessing learning in school
- developing strategies for emotional regulation or social skills, improving integration at school
- assessing for and providing specialist equipment, e.g. supportive seating, promoting function
- adapting tasks and environment to match the child/young person's abilities, e.g. ramp provision for access in and out of the home
- interventions preventing contractures after severe burns
- task and activity analysis for children/young people with arthritis, advising how task adaptations can save energy and strain on joints.

If working for the NHS you may provide a specialist assessment of the child/young person's level of skill and functional ability across a number of performance areas, for example assessing manipulation skills and the impact of any challenges including use of fastenings whilst dressing, use of cutlery when eating and pencil or cutting skills at school. NHS occupational therapists also assess for, and recommend, specialist equipment including supportive seating.

(Note: Many authorities have wanted to integrate their health and social care paediatric occupational therapy teams, but there are obstacles including separate IT systems. If you work in an integrated team I recommend you also read Chapter 9.)

What do I need to know as a paediatric occupational therapist?

Where do we start? What areas of practice and therapeutic interventions do we need to know about?

Child-related legislation
Common childhood conditions
Safeguarding
Models of practice
Knowledge base underpinning paediatric occupational therapist
Roles and responsibilities of other child care professionals
Child-centred practice
Moving and handling
Frames of reference – paediatrics

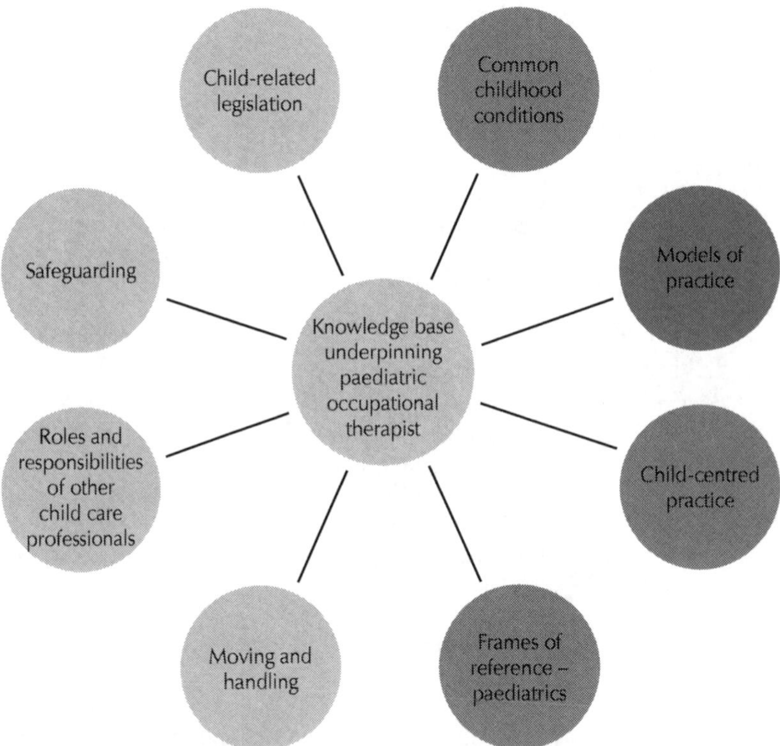

Figure 5.1 Areas of paediatric practice
Source: Melanie Elliott

This chapter will focus on the areas on the right hand side of Figure 5.1, but other chapters provide information on many of the other areas.

Frames of reference and models of practice

Frames of reference (FoR) within occupational therapy draw on a range of sciences to support and inform clinical application influencing practice, including:

- developmental theories

- learning theories
  - cognitive sciences
  - behaviourism
  - neurosciences
  - motor learning
- motor control and human movement sciences.

You will have covered many FoRs at university, but not necessarily learned to apply them to new areas of practice. (In my experience, you often begin by familiarising yourself with service and team protocols, criteria, day-to-day working practices and assessment and interventions; essential, but don't forget FoR.)

If you have no prior paediatric knowledge you are expected to complete some self-study on child development at the very least. You will be mentored and supported, ensuring you have gathered information you need, then supported in analysing this to identify and prioritise identified challenges. Initially you may need support developing your intervention plans; if you are unsure always ask. On a case-by-case base you will find new situations and invariably things you don't know – this is a positive, you can then learn about these, thereby progressing your professional development.

There are skills requiring formal training courses to bring you up to speed. Some are one- or two-day courses, others longer postgraduate courses. (Note: If employed by statutory services, large charities or private companies there is core mandatory training for you as a professional representing and providing services on behalf of your employer. Safeguarding, for example will be covered wherever you work.)

There is a huge amount of information to take on board. Below is a brief overview to assist you in organising knowledge you will use. With experience you will begin put it all together in your day-to-day practice without thinking about each area separately. In other words, your practice will be truly child-centred as you automatically apply what is relevant and necessary to their needs and circumstances. You will continue to build and expand your knowledge base and experience throughout your career.

Models of practice

Models have been covered extensively during your training. However, it is worth re-capping. Mosey identifies models of practice as a profession's 'fundamental body of knowledge' (cited in Turpin and Iwama 2010, p.18). Knowledge describing philosophy and theory, including relevant scientific data, underpins our profession.

Models explain the purpose of occupational therapy as a profession – what we do, why we do it, what we achieve by doing it, setting out evidence from scientific data, legitimising theory and philosophy, dealing with professional identity as a whole.

They also describe 'a domain of concern and legitimate tools' (Turpin and Iwama 2010, p.18) guiding the way you conceptualise practice and communicate your role and support the ongoing development of our profession.

Frames of reference (FoR)

An FoR is the working knowledge/'applied knowledge' (Mosey, cited in Turpin and Iwama 2010, p.18), guiding day-to-day application of knowledge, bridging theory and practice.

FoRs:

- set out *theory* and then describe what this *means/how it is relevant* in day-to-day practice with children/young people and families
- detail *therapeutic intervention techniques/approaches* developed as a result of the theory
- *set standards* for practice and provide agreed and shared terminology for the application for an intervention
- set out means of *evaluating* both application and impact of techniques
- *evidence* practical applications using research from the field of occupational therapy and other related fields of study
- enable therapists to explain interventions to children/young people/parents/carers or education/residential settings (Berry and Ryan 2002).

Below are a few of the most common FoRs in paediatric occupational therapy:

- developmental
- occupational behaviour
- biomechanical
- neurodevelopmental
- sensory integration
- motor learning
- visual perception.

Each FoR has a specific focus, such as increasing social participation or handwriting. As therapists you are not confined to a single FoR. Frequently therapists are eclectic in choice and application, each offering slightly different strategies and interventions. Being truly child-centred frequently sees therapists using a combination of interventions from different FoRs, tailoring interventions to the child/young person's needs.

Using multiple FoRs is similar to having a variety of implements/tools, you choose the one most suited to needs identified by your assessment; often you will use more than one frame of reference at a time. Completing a good assessment is key.

Not every FoR relevant to paediatric occupational therapy has been covered, this is merely an introduction. (To find out more about the social participation and acquisitional frames of reference, see recommended reading.)

RECOMMENDED READING

P. Kramer and J. Hinojosa (2010) *Frames of Reference for Pediatric Occupational Therapy*, 3rd edn. Hagerstown, MD: Lippincott Williams and Wilkins.

Developmental frame of reference

This is not a FoR in the true sense of the word, as it does not prescribe means of evaluation or intervention. It can be considered the foundation upon which we carry out assessment and intervention planning.

There is an enormous amount of information available on child development, as it is of interest to and relevant for all educators, education establishments, policy makers, paediatricians, medical personal, clinical and educational psychologists, physiotherapists, speech and language therapists, play therapists and so on, all drawing on and contributing to this body of knowledge. It can be a challenge to decide where to start and how much to learn.

As an occupational therapist you will need an idea of skills a child/young person is expected to have gained for their age, providing some comparison to the typically developing population. An understanding of stages of child development, their sequence and approximate timings is essential to assess a child/young person, providing an idea of what you may expect to see at a moment in time. This assists identification of developmental deficits and challenges requiring additional support/intervention. You must then consider the impact of any delays or difficulties on the child/young person's ability to function, participate socially or engage in activities of their choosing.

The developmental FoR also informs your intervention planning, enabling setting of developmentally appropriate goals and/or making appropriate adaptations to either task or environment.

The simplified example below illustrates the use of multiple FoRs but primarily emphasises how dependent you are on a good foundation in development.

> You work with a child with a physical disability who has not yet developed independent sitting as expected to do so given their age (*developmental* FoR). This holds back their hand function, eye–hand coordination and feeding. You use the *biomechanical* FoR to address postural control and core stability so they can sit up and access play with their hands. You also identify which skills they need to develop in terms of hand function (*developmental* FoR; your expectation based on age-appropriate abilities). You may not target age-appropriate skills straight away, instead you may have to address steps missed in development of manipulation, but at least the developmental FoR has given you direction.

Remember 'normal' development is variable. Traditionally theories focused on linear progression, that is, milestones, biased towards genetics being responsible for development. Now there are multiple theories taking into account many influences on a child's development such as environment, opportunities and nurturing.

RECOMMENDED READING

A. Sharma and H. Cockerill (2014) *Mary Sheridan's from Birth to Five Years: Children's Developmental Progress*, 4th edn. Abingdon: Routledge, Taylor & Francis.

M. Sheridan (2010) *Play in Early Childhood*, 3rd edn, rev. J. Howard and D. Alderson. Abingdon: Routledge Taylor & Francis.

J. Case-Smith and J. Clifford O'Brien (2014) *Occupational Therapy for Children and Adolescents*, 7th edn. Maryland Heights, MS: Elsevier Mosby.

C. Meggitt (2012) *Child Development: An Illustrated Guide: Birth to 19 Years*. Harlow: Pearson Education.

Functional/occupational behaviour

Understanding occupation and use of occupation as therapy are corner stones of the occupational therapy profession. Like the developmental FoR this a conceptual approach forming part of our foundation for assessment and intervention.

Play, learning, social interaction and developing independence are childhood occupations. A person's interests, values, skills, roles, habits and goals influence their choice of occupation/activity and determine their occupational behaviour. Applied to children, their interests, likes, dislikes, personalities, abilities, biology, support and opportunities drive their exploration and play. Successful exploration and positive experiences are repeated and thus children grow and develop through active participation. What they like, value and choose to do affects their occupational behaviour.

There are a number of occupation-based theoretical models but in paediatric occupational therapy the Person–Environment–Occupation–Performance (PEOP) model is most frequently cited. This model, with others, contributes to the Synthesis of Child, Occupational, Performance and Environment-In Time (SCOPE-IT)

FoR referred to by Kramer and Hinojosa (2010). This model aims to develop a child's occupational performance through 'maximization of the child-environment fit' (p.272).

When we assess a child/young person we look for their challenges and strengths. We look at the environment in which they live and function – what opportunities for participation and independence are there? Last, but not least, we need to consider their personality, self-esteem, cognitive ability, age and stage of development. Analysis of the information assists with developing an intervention strategy using their strengths, interests and motivation, whilst also looking at the context in which we expect them to function, making changes or adaptations where necessary.

Therapists frequently use assessment tools such as School Function Assessment, the Assessment of Motor and Process Skills (AMPS) and the Pediatric Evaluation of Disability Inventory (PEDI) to look at things specific to the child influencing occupational performance. These are used as part of a holistic assessment. Understanding what is important and motivating for the child is critical in helping us plan interventions. It does not matter how brilliant your intervention plan looks on paper, or how creative and skill specific your therapeutic activities are, if they are of no interest or relevance to the child/young person they will not be effective. We need to present/suggest or provide support enabling them to do things they want and need to do because they are *meaningful*, *relevant* and *important* to *them*. Remember occupational performance is the means *and* the end; we use occupations to develop skills *and* we develop skills to enhance occupation.

Biomechanical

The biomechanical FoR considers aspects such as range of motion (ROM), endurance, strength and posture. In paediatric occupational therapy it forms the basis for interventions addressing joint contractures, posture and proximal stability for distal function, where there is impairment of musculoskeletal or neuromuscular functions.

It is frequently used for children/young people with physical disability, understanding impacts of deficits on a child's biomechanics and function is critical; how does posture impact on feeding, toileting, hand function and ability to move from one position to another, and so on? You would use the biomechanical FoR in combination with functional/occupational behaviour FoR and developmental FoR to link physical and performance challenges. It offers visible and measurable outcomes.

Biomechanical intervention usually takes the form of specialist equipment to achieve optimal positions for participation and function whilst reducing the risk of postural deformity and asymmetry, including:

- *specialist, supportive seating* enabling children to develop hand function and feeding skills
- *sleep systems,* used primarily for comfort and positioning at night (a number of specialist equipment companies offer sleep systems – your department will have guidance for assessment and monitoring of these as children are constantly growing and changing. Regular review to check size and fit is essential, occupational therapy teams often have review systems in place)
- *upper limb splinting* using static thermoplastic or semi-dynamic neoprene splints is another good example of the application of this FoR. (You need to be taught to make and/or choose appropriate splints, often there are team members with these skills keeping up to date with developments in practice. Once again, clear user instructions and regular review are essential.)

> A child/young person with cerebral palsy has developed an elbow contracture resulting from hypertonicity. The medical consultant provides a course of Botox to relax the muscles and release the contracture. Occupational therapists in acute settings will work alongside the consultant, providing a thermoplastic splint to sustain muscle stretch following Botox treatment. This splint is remoulded regularly to increase ROM at the elbow using a goniometer to measure the joint angle at each stage.

Neurodevelopmental (NDT)

This approach focuses on understanding neuromuscular dysfunction, that is, poor motor control, atypical muscle tone, atypical movement patterns, postural difficulties and so on, and is also known as 'Bobath Therapy' after its originators Berta and Karl Bobath.

This FoR has its basis in neuroscience, motor control, motor learning and human movement science relying on the presence of neuroplasticity. NDT requires postgraduate training, following a period of clinical experience with individuals with neuromuscular dysfunction, for example cerebral palsy, brain injury and stroke. Information about courses can be found at www.bobath.org.uk.

Intervention involves hands-on therapeutic handling, a dynamic interaction between the child/young person and therapist. The therapist uses their knowledge of typical and atypical movement patterns to facilitate and guide functional movement patterns, whilst inhibiting undesirable patterns of movement.

This FoR is used in combination with the biomechanical FoR as well as the developmental and occupational performance FoR. It provides therapy targeting changes in motor control but children often have specialist equipment and/or are advised on fun, playful activities to support work done in therapy sessions.

An example of the above-mentioned FoRs at work together:

> A child with cerebral palsy attends regular therapy sessions with an NDT trained therapist working on upper limb movement. They work towards establishing a pattern of movement enabling the child to independently bring a loaded spoon to their mouth. Being able to feed themselves is important to them and their family (*developmental and occupational behaviour* FoR). The therapist will ensure they have supportive seating assisting with postural alignment (*biomechanical* FoR) also considering the task and tools, possibly providing eating utensils with enlarged grip and/or a plate with a raised lip keeping food contained on the plate (*occupational behaviour* FoR – SCOPE-IT).

Sensory integration (SI)

As with NDT, sensory integration requires postgraduate training. Jean Ayres developed the theory of SI over a number of years, beginning in the 1950s (Ayres 2005). The theory hypothesises sensory information from the environment and within the body is automatically and unconsciously processed, organised and integrated by the brain so we respond in a timely and appropriate manner to what is happening around us. Difficulties processing and integrating information impact on performance, as information on which we base actions is inaccurate.

The foundations for treatment lie in neuroscience (Lane and Schaaf 2010), and there is an emerging evidence base for the efficacy of this intervention (May-Benson and Koomar 2010; Miller, Coll and Schoen 2007; Pfeiffer *et al.* 2011; Schaaf *et al.* 2012, 2013). Neuroscience provides evidence that sensory input, or sensory and/or opportunity rich environments, combined with movement can influence brain structure and function (Lane and Schaaf 2010).

This FoR describes/explains why emotional, functional, social, motor coordination, attention and concentration difficulties can arise from poor assimilation and integration of sensory information. Therapists are taught how to assess for and treat SI difficulties. There are clear treatment principles and fidelity measures to ensure these principles are adhered to. Goal setting is taught to therapists trained in SI to help with evaluation SI therapy. Research is ongoing, evidence for this FoR drawn from neuroscience occupational therapy case studies and trials.

What does SI look like in practice?

Once a child has been fully assessed using a range of assessment tools and found to have sensory processing difficulties, they may be given a block of Ayres Sensory Integration (ASI) therapy. These are one-to-one sessions, the child and therapist in a room containing a range of activity opportunities including access to suspended equipment such as platform swings. From an observer's point of view it appears the child is playing and the therapist is joining in. It is important the play is child led – but the therapist will have chosen and laid out specific, suitable activities prior to sessions offering activities most beneficial to the child. During the sessions the therapist continually scaffolds, adapts and extends activities to provide the '*just right*' challenge. The therapist observes closely and responds to the child, seeing when and how to maximise the child's opportunities to adapt to challenges within play, as self-initiated movement is powerful in laying down new neural pathways. The 'just right' challenge stretches the child slightly, but is achievable, so they experience success and are motivated to repeat activities; repetition helps to lay down new neural pathways, in doing so enabling new skill acquisition.

Recent research finds two to three sessions a week for shorter blocks of therapy are effective. Not all statutory services are able to provide this intensive treatment due to limited resources. However, there are a growing number offering training on sensory processing difficulties to families and/or schools, empowering them to consider children's sensory needs and to make task and/or environmental changes to meet these or change daily routine. Such changes and adaptations are *not* to be confused with ASI.

This is an example of adaptations based on an understanding of sensory processing:

> A child is unable to sit still and focus in class, constantly moving. The teacher may recognise this as a true sensory need for movement and provide an air-filled cushion to sit on during lessons and carpet-time so they are moving but remain in place. They may also incorporate a whole class five-minute physical exercise programme at the beginning of the day, mid-morning or after lunch. In addition, they may ask the child to run errands (e.g. taking the register to the office or handing out pencils), providing regular movement breaks.

As sensory processing issues gain recognition agencies have included these as possible contributing factors to presenting challenges. Whilst many occupational therapists and other professional groups are not necessarily trained to deliver ASI, they may make recommendations for task or environmental modifications considering the child/young person's sensory processing challenges.

The Sensory Integration Network UK and Ireland website (www.sensoryintegration.org.uk) is informative and easy to use, giving information on how to pursue study in SI and its application.

Motor learning theory

How do we learn and acquire movement skills? There are many theories on motor learning. The one most applied in occupational therapy is the dynamic systems theory developed by Esther Thelen (Case-Smith and Clifford O'Brien 2014), a developmental theory concerned with how new behaviours originate.

This theory proposes we naturally seek solutions to new and unfamiliar tasks. Solutions to new tasks depend on the nature of the task, children's personal attributes, existing skills and previous experience, biology and the environment in which they find themselves. It recognises the dynamic interplay between child–environment–task: the child's skills cannot be viewed in isolation.

Environments are unpredictable and changing, providing different learning circumstances; equally tasks can be different for multiple reasons. It offers opportunities for therapists to use constraints/controls in either environment or task to influence the child's response.

The Cognitive Orientation to Daily Occupational Performance (CO-OP) draws on motor learning theory. In paediatrics, motor learning principles have been used most often with developmental coordination disorder and cerebral palsy. The child/young person is trained to monitor their performance and consciously evaluate the quality and outcome.

RECOMMENDED READING

A. Mandich and H. Polatajko (2004) *Enabling Occupation in Children: The Cognitive Orientation to Daily Occupational Performance (CO-OP) Approach*. Ottawa, ON: CAOT Publications ACE.

From Zwicker and Harris (2009) and others we see the principles of motor learning theory focus on:

- stages of learning: cognitive, associative and autonomous
- types of tasks: discrete, continuous, open or closed
- practice: massed, distributed, blocked, random, part versus whole
- feedback: extrinsic or intrinsic, timing – concurrent, immediate, terminal
- knowledge of results and performance.

Visual perception

Visual perception is more than the ability to see, it is the ability to *interpret* and *understand* what you see, enabling you to make sense of what you see, guiding movement when learning new skills. Visual information is not processed in isolation but integrated with all other sense inputs; however, you need to be able to pick up visual information before you begin to process it. For this you need vision and occulo-motor control. Often families will already have visited an optometrist to check a child's visual acuity and field. Remember to ask if they have been prescribed glasses before proceeding with any further assessment.

(It is helpful to familiarise yourself with the remit of a behavioural optometrist so you can signpost families should you identify any occulo-motor issues. These are optometrists with a particular interest in the impact of vision on day-to-day performance.)

A child/young person with visual perceptual difficulties could present with:

- poor visual attention
- difficulty recognising, sorting and matching objects (finding toys in a box, clothing items in a drawer, unable to sort clothes by type or identify matching socks)
- problems retaining visual information which negatively affect written communication and ability to follow written instructions
- issues organising letters/numbers on a page, moving around in unfamiliar spaces, judging depth of steps/noticing changes in floor surfaces, playing as part of a team, knowing where you need to be in relation to team members, bumping into objects
- difficulties copying letters, numbers or drawings
- challenged by basic self-care activities (fastening buttons, putting toothpaste on a toothbrush, combing or brushing hair).

As occupational therapists we assess visual perception by gathering a comprehensive history and description of presenting problems, completing observations in familiar settings and use of standardised assessments including:

- TVPS-4-Test of Visual Perceptual Skills
- Developmental Test of Visual Perception
- Beery-Buktenica Developmental Test of Visual-Motor Integration.

Further reading is recommended, putting your day-to-day learning of assessment and intervention into the wider context. For example, when you are taught how to administer the Movement ABC or the Test of Visual Perceptual Skills it will help you to understand theory underpinning these, and where they fit into the scheme of things.

- Why are you assessing this skill?
- What do the results mean?
- What intervention options are there?
- How does this translate into day-to-day living for the child/ young person or family?

Note: Visual perception has a significant impact on reading and writing and as a result you are likely to be using the assessments listed above when assessing handwriting.

Handwriting draws from multiple frames of reference for assessment and intervention. There is a wealth of information and resources available including from the National Handwriting Association and regular, occupational therapist-specific training courses.

Child/family-centred practice

Actively involving children and families in the assessment and intervention planning process is key to client-centred practice, requiring occupational therapists to address occupations most meaningful to the child/young person and family. This approach involves them in goal setting, eliciting motivations and commitment, allowing for routine-based interventions; those set within the natural/normal environments and embedded within everyday family routines and activities ensuring skills are both functional and meaningful.

A child needs to develop bilateral upper limb coordination. The occupational therapist looks at activities they would normally do at home/school or other care settings, working with parents/educators or carers to identify tasks and activities providing opportunities for developing this skill.

They enjoy cooking/baking. It's helpful to give them tasks such as grating, mixing, rolling to do, as these inherently require use of both hands together. You may need to help parents/carers to:

- break the task down, e.g. roll out ready-made pastry to start with, later progressing to rolling out a larger ball of pastry
- adapt the task, e.g. use a large handled spoon for stirring with non-slip matting under the mixing bowl, preventing it from sliding around while the child practises stabilising it with one hand
- gradually build up levels of challenge to develop ongoing improvements in coordination.

It is a collaborative approach, maintaining the family's natural rhythm and daily routine, sensitive to the uniqueness of each child/young person and family, acknowledging parents/carers know their child best and want what is best for their child.

RECOMMENDED READING

D. Jennings, M.F. Hanline and J. Woods (2012) 'Using routines-based interventions in early childhood special education.' *Dimensions of Early Childhood 40*, 2, 13–23.

Assessments

In paediatrics the assessment process is similar to other areas of practice, however parent/carer participation is essential. As outlined in the child/family-centred practice section, there is child–parent interaction to consider, as well as the impact of a child's needs/challenges on families as a whole.

Environments differ, frequently home/nursery/school, a child's occupations being play and learning. Finally, one must look at self-care/independence skills depending on age.

Figure 5.2 summarises how information can be gathered. Self-report should always be considered, it is important to obtain the child/young person's view. There are assessments available to support this, such as the Child Occupational Self-Assessment v 2.2, Self-Image Profiles (SIP) and the Conner's Comprehensive Behavior Rating Scales (CBRS) which include a self-report section.

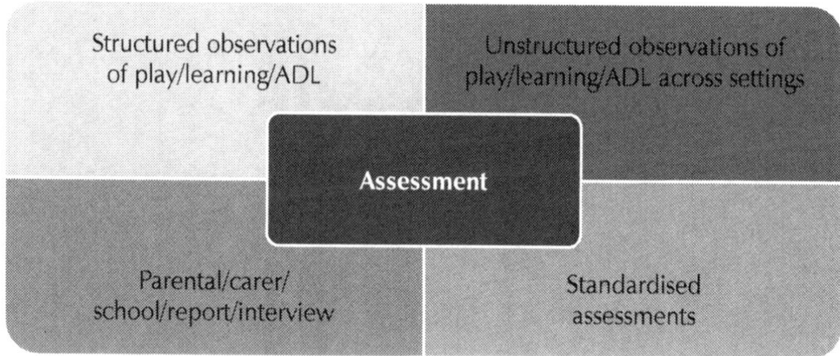

Figure 5.2 Types and locations of assessments
Source: Melanie Elliott

Standardised assessments

You will already be familiar with standardised tests and their importance clinically. Departments will have standardised assessments best suiting their client group, timescales in which to complete assessments, service remits, knowledge and skills of assessing therapists and budget limits. Therefore each has slightly different resources with regard to assessment tools.

Some tests are used as *screening tools*, typically taking 20–30 minutes to administer, assisting identification of individuals needing further assessment/input. Others are used for more in-depth assessments of developmental skills, function, cognition and social domains. It is important you take time to familiarise yourself with available tests and to practise administering them. The key to standardisation is *uniformity in administration* and scoring *between and by* all therapists.

EXAMPLES OF COMMONLY USED SCREENING TOOLS
Sensory Processing Measure (SPM)
Miller Assessment of Pre-schoolers (MAP)
Movement Assessment Battery for Children – 2nd edition (Movement ABC-2)

EXAMPLES OF MORE IN-DEPTH ASSESSMENTS
Bruininks-Oseretsky Test of Motor Proficiency – 2nd edition (BOT-2)
Sensory Integration and Praxis Test (SIPT)

This is not a definitive list of assessments. The ones listed are examples only.

Websites of companies supplying standardised assessments in the UK are listed below, most with area representatives with test examples for you to look at and to answer queries:

- www.pearsonclinical.co.uk
- www.annarbor.co.uk
- www.winslowresources.com
- www.hogrefe.co.uk

Note: Assessing for specialist equipment is not part of your initial assessment. It is an action *arising* from an identified need in your initial assessment. Remember to work within the parameters of your service. Initially see if there are suitable items of stock equipment already available to you. If not, research options, then contact respective companies requesting a joint visit with the equipment you would like to try. The equipment representative will be able to *advise* you on features and possible adaptations for items in order to meet the child's need. It is *your responsibility* to assess if equipment appropriately meets the need.

Paediatric occupational therapy process

You are familiar with the occupational therapy assessment process. Figure 5.3 is not intended as a teaching tool but as a reminder with pointers to recall while you are still learning; eventually this process will be automatic.

Reason/ Referral	What are the issues/challenges facing the child/young person? What are the concerns? What is the impact on their function?
Gathering Background Information	Gathering background information through assessing shared/historic records with consent (usually gained at the point of referral). It is helpful to familiarise yourself with any diagnosis or condition relating to the child/young person.
Preparing for the Appointment	You will see the child/young person in their home/in clinic/in school or college. Make sure the address and contact details for the visit are accurate. Appointments can be arranged by telephone or letter. Confirm appointments before going, especially in the community and going a long way. Follow the department's procedures for lone working if out in the community.
Parent/ Carer Interview	Make sure you are familiar with any information already shared by the family with colleagues in other professions to avoid repetition. To begin with you may find it helpful to use a questionnaire to become familiar with and accustomed to the type of information most helpful to you. Often there are existing assessment forms within your service. This information is part of your assessment.
Assessment	You can use a range of tools – checklists, questionnaires, standardised assessments, clinical observations, observations in different environments and/or play. You may need more than one session to complete an assessment depending on the reason for the assessment, e.g. for seating you may want to look at more than one option.
Treatment/ Intervention Plan	To reach this stage you have to analyse the information you have gathered so far to identify the main issues from an occupational therapy perspective. This should be done in collaboration with the child/young person and their family. You may identify learning to tie shoelaces as a target, but if parents are unconcerned by this and are happy to provide Velcro fastening shoes instead, there is little point in pursuing this. Your treatment plan outlines what you are going to do. It is often multi-faceted and requires the use of a range of occupational therapy skills, therapeutic tools and approaches.

Figure 5.3 Paediatric occupational therapy process
Source: Melanie Elliott

Treatment

By analysing assessment data you will identify areas to be addressed to support the child/young person and their family. (Sometimes there are issues outside your professional area of expertise. In this case signposting, or referring, the family to appropriate services is identified as an objective in your intervention plan.)

As an occupational therapist you are looking to support development, skill acquisition, participation and function. Promoting safe manual handling and supporting and enabling good posture, symmetry and alignment may be part of this.

How you do this is often through a combination of the approaches as summarised in Figure 5.4.

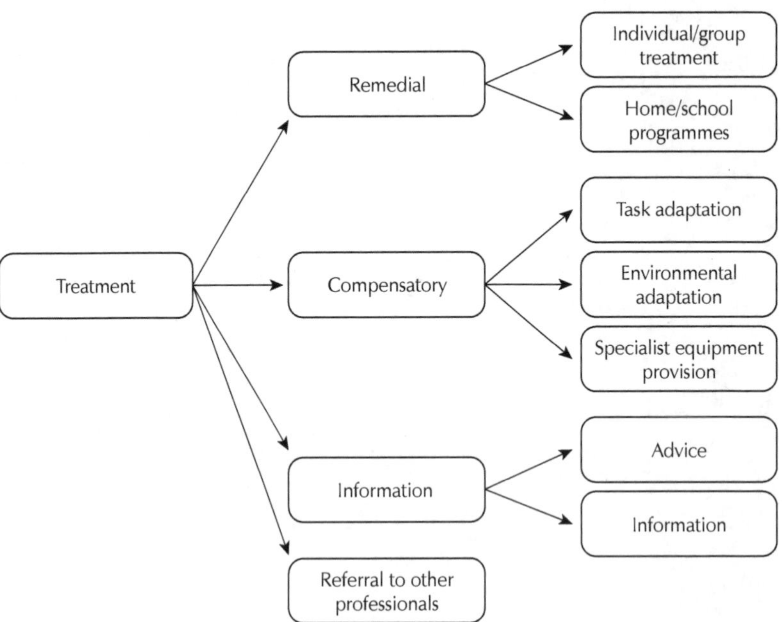

Figure 5.4 Paediatric occupational therapy approaches
Source: Melanie Elliott

> An example is a child/young person who presents with handwriting difficulties. You identified visual perceptual difficulties and noted visual pursuits are not smooth. You also identified poor pencil grip and reduced shoulder stability. (Your analysis will probably be far more in depth; this illustration is simplified.)

Your action plan may look something like this:

- *Refer* to behavioural optometry for investigation of difficulties with visual pursuits. (Parental consent is *essential*, especially as this is often pursued privately.)
- Trial different pencil grips encouraging more efficient grip, reducing cramping and improving control (*compensatory task adaptation*).
- Check desk and chair height in the classroom are correct for writing following ergonomic principles (*environmental adaptation*).
- Address shoulder girdle stability through PE activities and play activities at home (*remedial – home and school programme*).
- Discuss with the teacher classroom strategies to reduce the impact of identified visual perceptual difficulties (*advice and information*).

Occupational therapists working in paediatrics regularly visit and work collaboratively with teachers and teaching assistants, contributions frequently captured in a child's *education, health and care plans* (EHC plans). These capture input from all professionals involved with a child, aiming to coordinate actions, ensuring aims and objectives are holistic. EHC plans lay out clearly resources each agency will provide for the child/young person and provide a means of monitoring and capturing progress and/or change.

Common childhood conditions

The purpose of this section is not to describe the presenting symptoms, prognosis and occupational/functional implications of commonly occurring childhood conditions. It aims to identify conditions most prevalent and worthy of focused attention as you begin your paediatric career. Listed below are conditions you are most likely to find in day-to-day practice.

- Cerebral palsy
- Autism spectrum disorder (ASD)

- Down's syndrome
- Attention deficit hyperactivity disorder and attention deficit disorder
- Developmental coordination disorder
- Acquired brain injury
- Handwriting difficulties
- Feeding difficulties.

Note: Sensory processing disorder has not been listed, although it can be a discrete diagnosis. Sensory processing issues, however, frequently co-exist with other diagnoses. For example, *The Diagnostic and Statistical Manual of Mental Disorders* (American Psychiatric Association 2013) now includes atypical sensory processing as a diagnostic feature for ASD (Smith Roley *et al.* 2015).

You will always be faced with conditions new to you, requiring self-directed learning when you first become involved. Knowing where to access information and who to contact is important. The charity Contact a Family provide information, advice and support to families, facilitating contact between families and local and national support groups where children share a diagnosis or similar challenges. They also provide online chat facilities for parents and advice on education and children's services. They have a comprehensive list of conditions relevant to paediatrics and provide support and training to professionals working with children and young people.

Professional specialist interest groups

You may join professional specialist interest groups accessible through the Royal College of Occupational Therapists (RCOT) website to further your knowledge. They provide access to the national network of occupational therapists working in paediatrics, peer-reviewed journals, research support, advice, continuing professional development (CPD) opportunities and access to clinical forums. Initially RCOT SS-Children, Young People and Families would be most helpful. Later specialisation may be supported through membership of People with Learning Disabilities, Housing, Mental Health or Occupational Therapists in Private Practice.

Safeguarding training

This is mandatory and provided by your employer; training supports learning about safeguarding children and young people, also guiding you through the reporting process. Each organisation has clear pathways guiding you in raising concerns you may have about a child/young person you are involved with.

> If you are self-employed you will need to seek this training independently.
>
> The National Society for the Prevention of Cruelty to Children (NSPCC) provide an online training course: www.nspcc.org.uk/what-you-can-do/get-expert-training/child-protection-schools-online-course.

Manual handling

This is mandatory training if you are working with physical disability and/or equipment provision and/or home adaptations. Once again, your employer provides you with training, teaching you about safe techniques and an introduction to equipment including hoists, slings and slide sheets. You may have completed this at university but your employer has a duty to ensure you remain safe in your practice. *If you are in private practice you will have to source this training independently.* A large number of providers can be found on the internet.

Each year there are specialist equipment exhibitions providing therapists with opportunities to see and learn about equipment including hoists, slings, slide sheets, lifting equipment and so on. Attend if you can. It is a great way to familiarise yourself with equipment and make contact with representatives of equipment companies. Look out for adverts in professional journals and join mailing lists so you know when, and where, exhibitions will be.

Other child care professionals

During training you will have worked alongside, and possibly shared lectures with, other allied healthcare disciplines and may understand their core roles. However, as with occupational therapy, there will be areas of specialisation by other professionals working within paediatrics. When you begin your new job your manager will probably have an induction period in mind. Some departments will arrange meetings for you, others leave it to you to arrange visits and identify relevant learning. If this is the case, try to spend time with the other disciplines within the wider multi-disciplinary team. This provides insight into their role, the structure of their service and how to access it if necessary.

If you identify a concern through your assessment outside your area of expertise the knowledge of other services is key to your ability to appropriately refer a child/young person to the necessary service and/or signpost families.

Courses and training

Your employer provides mandatory training, additional training is dependent on service needs, funding and staffing. You will need to discuss courses you are interested in, or have identified as relevant, with your supervisor or line manager. If they are in agreement, there are usually study leave and funding application processes to follow.

You will find information on courses in *OT News*, through specialist interest section membership, the OT magazine or on websites such as the Sensory Integration Network UK and Ireland website.

Occupational therapy events are great learning and networking opportunities too, so consider exhibitions, both locally and nationally, and remember the RCOT's library services and electronic journals (found in the 'Practice Resources' section of the RCOT website) when searching for specific information.

Conclusion

To conclude, paediatric practice is an exciting field of occupational therapy to work in with many varied and interesting employment opportunities. Each child/young person is unique. What works for one may not work for another, despite presenting with similar diagnosis or difficulty. Being child-centred, working collaboratively with families and with other professions is challenging, effective and rewarding.

There is a real emphasis on further professional development and learning with a host of postgraduate training opportunities. The research and evidence base underpinning our practice is continuously growing and practice evolving. Occupational therapists have a unique skill set and much to offer with our focus on occupation and function. It is a *very* worthwhile journey.

USEFUL WEBSITES

American NDT Association for Professionals for the Advancement of NDT: www.ndta.org

British Association of Behavioural Optometrists: www.babo.co.uk

Contact a Family: https://cafamily.org.uk

CO-OP: www.co-opacademy.ca

National Handwriting Association: www.nha-handwriting.org.uk

OT Magazine: http://ot-magazine.co.uk

RCOT: www.rcot.co.uk

SEND: www.gov.uk/children-with-special-educational-needs/extra-SEN-help and www.ipsea.org.uk/what-you-need-to-know/ehc-plans

Sensory Integration Network UK and Ireland: www.sensoryintegration.org.uk

Task/environment modifications: www.autism.org.uk/environment

6

MENTAL HEALTH

Sara Brewin

Introduction

If you've picked up this book and are reading this chapter, I'm guessing you have possibly chosen, or are considering, working within an adult community mental health team (CMHT).

Before we start, you're probably wondering what qualifies me to advise you and write a chapter in a book! Well, I'm certainly no expert, and there are always new things to be learned, but I am qualified to share with you the knowledge and experience I have gained over the years in the hope that the start of your occupational therapy career in adult mental health won't be as daunting as it was for me.

Prior to beginning my occupational therapy training I worked as a community support worker within an adult CMHT. During this time, my supervision was carried out by an occupational therapist who inspired me to complete my occupational therapy qualification. It's been six years since I graduated and took up my first occupational therapy position within an adult CMHT. Though this was probably not quite as daunting as it would have been if I hadn't prior experience in this before my training, I was still pretty anxious about taking on this new role and hoping I would make a good occupational therapist. Now, I know what you're thinking, 'she already knows what she's doing': absolutely not. Although I had some experience of working within mental health I did not have experience or knowledge of working as an occupational therapist in a busy multi-disciplinary team (MDT).

I have always valued my role as an occupational therapist. It is unique but also diverse and allows us to think outside the box and be creative, as everyone is different and what might work for one does not work for all. However, like any role, it can sometimes be challenging, and I use my supervision sessions, professional and clinical, and liaise with peers and team members to explore options and see if I have missed something. Sometimes this extra input enables me to remain focused and move forward with the plan. The reward is achieving the outcome of getting someone to engage and begin working on their goals, supporting them in making positive changes, those being ones they have identified.

The chapter is written from my personal experience, which is why I shall illustrate one area of mental health, the role and interventions of occupational therapy within a CMHT for adults with a severe and enduring mental health difficulty. Although this is specific to one area of mental health, it is similar to and can encompass a wide range of other settings. This is completed by relating my current practice to the Royal College of Occupational Therapists (RCOT) *Code of Ethics and Professional Conduct* (2015) to demonstrate how I not only keep up to date with my practice and registration, but how the interventions delivered are person centred as well as within the *Recovering Ordinary Lives 2007–2017* strategy (College of Occupational Therapists 2006).

Note: Royal status was conferred on the College of Occupational Therapists in 2017. The original designation is therefore used for publications before that date.

Occupational therapy and mental health

As you are aware, the purpose of occupational therapy is to enable individuals to achieve, or work towards achieving, their identified goals by placing them at the centre of their care. The World Federation of Occupational Therapists (2010) statement supports this, and also states that occupational therapy enables the person to participate in activities of everyday life.

There are many definitions of mental health I have come across over the years and whilst doing the research for this chapter. However, the one which stands out for me comes from the World Health Organization, which defines mental health as 'a state of well-being in which individuals realise their own abilities, can cope with everyday stresses of life as well as working successfully and productively enabling them to contribute to their communities' (World Health Organization 2014).

Our role as occupational therapists is to assist people in maintaining or improving their functioning in order for them to achieve their identified goals. This is achieved by placing the person at the centre of their care and helping them to find or create opportunities to actively engage in activities/tasks as well as encouraging them to be more confident in making their own choices (College of Occupational Therapists 2006).

As an occupational therapist you need to ensure service users, carers and/or relatives have a clear understanding of your role, but this also applies to team members and other professionals and agencies. From personal experience, role confusion and a lack of understanding of occupational therapy is still present across many areas. However, strategies such as *Recovering Ordinary Lives 2007–2017* have been produced to help with clarity and understanding. But, as mentioned above, your role is to ensure you have a clear understanding of occupational therapy enabling promotion of our profession and the treatment and interventions we offer.

Occupational therapists also have roles within other mental health areas, which include acute in-patients, long-term mental health conditions, eating disorders and forensic settings as well as with child and adolescent mental health teams. Within different settings and teams the role of an occupational therapist can vary. However, the underlying role of the occupational therapist is placing the person at the centre of their care and assessing the person, their environment and occupations. Within assessments this can be broken down into self-care, productivity and leisure. This allows the occupational therapist to see the whole person and ensure nothing has been missed. If the occupational therapist has an understanding of the person they are working with, it allows the connection and trust to start to grow between the occupational therapist and individual, enabling a therapeutic relationship. The assessment also assists in identifying any current difficulties the person may be experiencing and areas they wish to change. This is where the person will begin to identify their goals with support and encouragement from the occupational therapist.

Working in a team

At the start of the chapter I mentioned working within a CMHT and a MDT. The CMHT is a team of health and social care workers who visit adults experiencing a severe and enduring mental health condition, generally within their own homes. The MDT is a varied team including the following roles:

- occupational therapists
- occupational therapy assistants
- peer support workers
- social workers
- social work assistants
- nursing assistants
- community psychiatric nurses (CPNs)
- Band 4 recovery practitioners (to aid in the recovery and discharge process)
- business support
- psychologists
- consultant psychiatrists.

All of these have an important and valued role within the team. I recommend that when you first start within CMHT you take opportunities to shadow all the different professionals, including your own. This will not only help you gain an understanding of the different roles but will also enable you to confidently identify if the person you are seeing requires interventions from another discipline in order to ensure they are receiving the most appropriate care and treatment.

Following on from the importance of team work, I'd like to briefly touch on inter-professional and inter-agency collaboration. This is described in an article by the Social Care Institute for Excellence (2009), the aim being to bring together service users, professionals, agencies, carers and service providers to work together to ensure the service delivered is person centred. Service users who you see may receive support and interventions from other agencies, if this is the case, clear communication is required considering confidentiality where necessary. I ensure I take a collaborative approach by recognising the need to work with, and alongside, other professionals and agencies. I do so by liaising using the most appropriate form of communication, for example face to face, email, telephone and, if necessary, jointly with the person, or independently, depending on the situation, as advised in the COT *Code of Ethics and Professional Conduct* (2015).

However, the most important thing to remember about team work is that *you are part of a team*, so if you're not sure of anything, ask! We've all been new to a position in our life and have needed help and guidance.

Getting started

So, first things first, policies and procedures. I know, not the most exciting start to your first day or week, but a very important requirement. These will be shown to you by the person doing your induction. Along with local policies and procedures, you may find it useful to look at *Recovering Ordinary Lives 2007–2017* (College of Occupational Therapists 2006). This is a strategy for occupational therapists working within mental health covering all areas of working practice across the four nations of the UK. The five themes that inform and shape the strategy are:

- valuing occupation
- education
- workforce development
- leadership
- added value of occupational therapy.

There is of course our code of ethics. However, I'm sure you don't need me to remind you (again) of the importance of adhering to it! Jokes aside, it is part of our professional agreement and, if we do experience a dilemma related to our professional or ethical conduct, it should be our first port of call, along with the support of colleagues.

Second, training. There is a variety of mandatory training to be completed on a regular basis. Most of it will be covered on your face-to-face trust induction. How training is presented will vary between face to face and online, depending on where you work, but it is compulsory in every trust. It is my advice that within mental health, the training priorities for you to focus on, and gain a great understanding of, are the Mental Health Act 1983, Mental

Capacity Act 2005, safeguarding, confidentiality, record keeping and risk. All the training is of equal importance and will enable you to continuously place the person at the centre of their care and meet our ethical standards.

Although not mandatory, but in my opinion just as important, accessing courses at local recovery colleges (if there are any in your area and if you are able to) is highly recommended for professional and personal benefits. I am involved with supporting our local recovery college, as I feel it can be very useful in providing opportunities for people to learn together, sharing experiences and knowledge. This enables people to gain further understanding and possible coping strategies around their own mental health, or about mental health in general. Because of this, I feel it is essential for new CMHT members to take recovery college learning opportunities, to help increase their awareness and so they can promote it to people they support.

Related legislation includes:

- Care Act 2014
- Data Protection Act 1998
- Equalities Act 2010, which incorporates the Disability Discrimination Act 1998
- Human Rights Act 1998
- National Health Service and Community Care Act 1990.

Third, prescription of equipment. Once you have joined the team I would suggest you enquire about completing the online training in order for you to receive a PIN which will allow you to order equipment via the Integrated Community Equipment Store (ICES). Occupational therapists within adult CMHTs hold a small budget in order to prescribe pieces of equipment to the people on their caseload if there is an assessed need. *This is only if you feel confident to do so.* Personally, I feel confident assessing for small items of equipment due to completing two placements where I observed and participated in assessing, measuring for and ordering equipment. However, I am aware of my limitations when it comes to a number of areas needing to be assessed. If it is not my area of expertise I ask a fellow occupational therapist or refer the person to adult social care, facilitating a full assessment of the person and identification of their needs.

Occupational therapy process

Referrals

Due to high demand for occupational therapy assessments a waiting list may be required to monitor referrals and ensure people are being assessed in turn. This was something which I felt was necessary for our team and which has made the process smoother as team members can access this for information. I would recommend starting one if you are swamped with referrals. Due to occupational therapy having a waiting list, I also find it good practice to send letters out to service users advising of the delay and suggesting they get in touch if they no longer require an assessment, or feel their situation has changed and an assessment is a higher priority than when they were first referred.

In order to ensure the occupational therapy process is focused around the person and their needs, the first step is the referral form. These short forms are compiled so the referrers can make a note of the person's name, date of birth, NHS number, reason for referral, referrer's information and date of referral. This allows the referrer to make the occupational therapist aware of any difficulties the person may have or any specific requirements the occupational therapist needs to meet. This means the person is assessed equally and fairly and in line with the Equality Act 2010 and relevant codes of ethics as well as allowing for reasonable adjustments to be made during the assessment or future interventions.

Within my trust once an occupational therapy referral is received (which can be made by any member of the CMHT), it is passed to Business Support for scanning onto our database and the hard copy placed in the referral folder for the occupational therapist to access. Best practice is for the referrer to have a face-to-face discussion with the occupational therapist so, during this conversation, the referrer can be made aware as to whether there is a waiting list. If this is not possible, you are required to search the database your team uses to find any appropriate information regarding the person. This will include notes, reviews, risk assessments and discussions with anyone currently or previously involved with the person, where possible. It is highly essential you document every step of your interventions and the contact you have with the person, whether it be written, face to face or through liaison with colleagues (where appropriate). This record starts from the moment you make initial contact with the person regarding an occupational therapy appointment. In line with the policy for the trust I work with regarding written notes, all contact has to be recorded within 24 hours of seeing, speaking with or liaising with/about the person and this record has to be both accurate and legible.

Assessment

A letter is sent out to the person offering an appointment at the base I work from to discuss possible occupational therapy interventions. Initial appointments are generally given at base if the person is new to the service (where risk can then be reviewed) or if there are any specific risks. However, if there is difficulty with accessing the team's base, a home visit can be planned. Following the initial assessment meeting, home visits are then generally carried out so the assessment can be completed in the person's home environment to allow for professional relationships to build. The aim of the initial meeting is for the occupational therapist to explain their role and give examples, where necessary, of previous interventions carried out by occupational therapy. It is also an opportunity for the person to discuss any difficulties they have or goals which they wish to work towards. This meeting allows the person and their carer, or family member if appropriate, to explore occupational therapy further and identify if they feel it is right for them to engage. At times people may not be ready to engage; it is essential this is recognised so people do not have a negative experience of occupational therapy, just because they were not in the right stage of their recovery to engage positively. If a person decides they are not ready to engage, or they don't feel it's appropriate, they are discharged back to their referrer who can re-refer in the future if required.

If a person is ready to engage a further appointment will then be given so an assessment can be completed and interventions can begin. The occupational therapy assessment mostly used within our trust, is the Model of Human Occupation Screening Tool.

Model of Human Occupation Screening Tool (MOHOST)

The MOHOST (Parkinson, Forsyth and Kielhofner 2006) is used to gather information relevant to the Model of Human Occupation concepts, which allow therapists to gain an overview of the person's occupational functioning. The aim of this screening tool is to capture the strengths the person has and to highlight the effects of volition (motivation for occupation), habituation (organisation), skills and the environment on a person's occupational performance. Completing this assessment with the person and carer, if this is appropriate, allows short- and long-term goals to be identified and placed in order of priority. Goals are planned by ensuring they are Specific, Measurable, Achievable, Realistic and Timed (SMART). This process is carried out alongside the person to ensure they are *their* goals.

The screening tool also identifies any specific difficulties the person may be experiencing, as well as identifying any reasonable adjustments need to be made in order to receive person-centred interventions. Because it is a thorough assessment lots of information can be gathered through conversation and through actively listening to the person, allowing them to identify changes they wish to make.

Fast track and discharge

Within the trust I work in, people who are ready to be discharged from the team can be placed on fast track. This is assessed on an individual basis as everyone's needs vary. If there is no need identified, then the person will be discharged back into the care of their GP with the person who referred them advised of the plan, if appropriate. If the person is placed on fast track, it means they can access the team for a set period of time, and do not have to be fully reassessed to access the team's support. Fast track is there to support people with their recovery, providing a safety net which will allow them to become more independent and gain confidence away from mental health services.

Groups

I'm sure you are well aware of the benefits of setting up and running groups within local communities and alongside community resources. Let me tell you about how, why and which groups are currently running with the community mental health team I work in.

In the past many groups were run by mental health workers, based at mental health sites. However, this has changed and many of the groups were unable to be supported by mental health teams. Despite this, anyone working in mental health knows the benefits and need for group work. With this in mind we began setting up groups at our base as well as in the local community. For the team I work in this included:

- emotional first aid (staff base)
- pool table group (within the community)
- carers' group (staff base)
- art group (staff base to begin with and then to be transferred to the community)
- recovery group (staff base).

These five groups are currently running and are successful, valued and well attended.

In order for groups to start up in the community and with local community services/businesses, collaborative working was key. For example, when setting up a cooking group I worked alongside a qualified chef (employed by the local council) delivering free cooking courses for a number of weeks. The success of this resulted in us being able to run the group again with just a small financial contribution.

I and the other occupational therapist in the team also worked alongside a local tennis club who offered (and still do) free tennis for any adult who has, or is experiencing, any mental health difficulty. The agreement with both groups was that a member of the local CMHT would be there for any mental health support required. This role has now been taken over by the occupational therapy assistant, who is employed within our team and is maintaining the positive relationship with the tennis club and supporting group members who attend.

The last group I would like to talk about is the carers' group. This was something I was keen to explore and set up, having worked with a variety of carers over the years who are not always able to attend a national organisation's carers' groups, or are without confidence to explore these. The first step was to identify carers on the team's caseloads and then providing information on a carers' group to be trialled once a week for six weeks. At the first meeting I explained to the group members I had not run a carers' group before but was aware there was a need for a local support group. Over the six weeks I shared information on community resources as well as other carer support which can be accessed. From the first week people began to engage and participate in group conversations, ranging from questions to seeking advice from other group members. On reviewing the six-week programme feedback was positive with one lady describing the group as a lifeline! This group is still running, now on a weekly basis for an hour and a half. Following this I have recently taken on the role as the carers' lead for my team, and I am looking forward to increasing the support available to carers.

So, if you have plans to start up a group, my advice is to make connections with your local community. Find out from people who access your service what they are interested in, or feel would be useful, and then promote it with your colleagues. Start a waiting list and then trial it. If the group can be moved in to the local community after the trial and eventually be peer run, with an occupational therapist or occupational therapy assistant supervising it monthly, this would be a positive step to people's recovery. As we are all aware, people do learn to manage their mental health and move forward from services. When and if this is the case, people may still want to access the groups they have been part of. This is why it is important to have groups based in local communities so they are still accessible.

Continuing professional development (CPD): A reflection

When first qualified as an occupational therapist I had great plans to maintain my CPD profile, and started off as I had been advised to as a student, guided by Health and Care Professions Council (HCPC) and RCOT codes of ethics and professional conduct. However, despite these great intentions, after about eight months of being in post the recording side of things slipped, for example, keeping a log of training and anything relating to my professional practice. I soon came to regret not keeping up with logging information. As I'm sure you're aware, there's a certain time of the year all healthcare professionals dread, and whether we will be chosen to provide evidence of our professional practice upon request from the HCPC.

So, in 2015 I was chosen. As I picked up the letter I knew what it wanted and then panic and regret set in. Luckily, working in the community I have a diary and if you work in the community your diary holds everything going on in your work life. This saved me. It had everything listed from training to student placements and meetings attended. Despite having this information, I then had the mammoth task of logging it all, asking for supportive letters from my team coordinator and a service user I had worked with, alongside collating all my reflective logs. This took time, *a lot of time*.

The advice I give is to keep a log of anything you do within your professional practice to evidence you are continuously up to date. This can be anything, including exploring other areas of practice to benefit service users, their carers and your team. Include any group work or supervision you deliver or receive, and training specific to your profession as well as generic training.

When writing my reflective pieces I used the Gibbs Reflective Cycle (Gibbs 1988), which has clear titles to follow, allowing a detailed description of the experience you are reflecting on. This enabled me to process my thoughts, give a clear description of the event, reflect and adapt for my future practice. There are many models out there, so explore them and find the one you relate to best.

Conclusion

The challenges of working within mental health vary from team to team, area to area. Resources and staffing are issues which always come up, no matter where you work.

If we think about it, it's pretty simple. Occupational therapists support and encourage individuals to identify what they would like to change, and support the individual to do so through identifying and setting realistic and achievable goals. This is accomplished by working collaboratively and, most of the time, thinking outside the box and being creative.

The benefits of working as an occupational therapist within mental health are rewarding: no matter how small the steps the individual you're working with takes, any step forward is a step closer to recovery and maintaining positive mental health. I'm not saying it's not challenging or difficult at times but, as I'm writing this, thoughts of people I have previously supported and those I am currently supporting pop in to my head and remind me why I love being an occupational therapist. I do my best and I hope that's enough to make small, positive changes in people lives, supporting them on their road to recovery. Now it's your turn.

Good luck!

7

LEARNING DISABILITIES

Ruth van der Weyden

Introduction

Welcome to the world of learning disabilities. This may be an area of occupational therapy you have experience in from being a student or from other work experience. Alternatively, you may be in a similar position to that I was in when I first qualified. As an occupational therapy student I had not completed any placements in learning disabilities, and my knowledge was only from my reading and what I had been taught at college.

I was very fortunate in having the opportunity to start my career working on a basic grade rotation, with my first post working in a learning disabilities team. For me, this is where it all started. I found the work stimulating, varied and rewarding. It enabled me to work as part of a team, utilising and developing a wide range of skills, using holistic and client-centred approaches.

The transition from being a student to starting a new job as a qualified occupational therapist can create different emotions: excitement, anticipation and, maybe, a little apprehension. In this chapter I draw from my own personal experience and point you in the direction of current literature and information which I think will help prepare and equip you to begin your career in learning disabilities.

What is a learning disability?

It is quite common for people to become confused between the terms *learning difficulty* and *learning disability*. This confusion can lead to people being referred to a learning disability team incorrectly, resulting in a need for signposting to an appropriate service.

A learning disability is a diagnosis, and is not just a descriptive term. According to the World Health Organization (1992, pp.225–231) the following three elements must all be present for a learning disability diagnosis to be made:

1. Incomplete or arrested development of the mind during childhood having a lasting effect on development.
2. A significant impairment of intellectual functioning, cognitive, language, motor, and social abilities; the person has an intelligence quotient (IQ) below 70.
3. A significant impairment of adaptive social functioning – this is where the person has a reduced ability to cope with daily activities, socialise and live independently. These are further defined as conceptual skills (communication, analysing information and problem solving), social skills and practical skills enabling a person to access the community, home living, self-care and work.

To make a diagnosis, a developmental history, intelligence tests (IQ tests) and assessments of social functioning are needed. Adaptive social functioning can be assessed using standardised assessments such as the Adaptive Behaviour Assessment Schedule or the Vineland. In some cases, the Assessment of Motor and Process Skills (AMPS) may also be used to aid assessment and diagnosis (Dwyer and Reep 2008).

AMPS is a standardised occupational therapy assessment. According to Mesa *et al.* (2014) 'Occupational Therapists can use the AMPS process competence cut-off of 1.0 logit to screen for "significant impairment of social and adaptive function" for learning disability diagnostic criteria' (p.173). Their article is informative about the use of AMPS in this way, and is well worth reading!

A person who has a learning disability will find it more difficult and take longer to understand new information and to develop new skills, and has difficulties with social communication. There are varying degrees of learning disability – mild, moderate, severe and profound. This will have an impact on the support a person needs with daily activities.

It is important to remember that although a learning disability is a diagnosis it is not an illness or disease. Northfield (cited in Goodman, Hurst and Locke 2009, p.2) suggests the term learning disability provides a label but does not describe the individuality of the person.

Health needs of people with a learning disability

There are many health conditions associated with having a learning disability. These can lead to or increase a person's risk of developing additional physical and mental health issues. For example, people with Down's syndrome can have congenital heart problems, a higher risk of developing Alzheimer's disease and a higher risk of gastrointestinal problems and cancer (Holland *et al.* 1998, cited in Michael 2008).

People who have profound and multiple learning disability often have postural care needs, increasing their risks of bowel and respiratory problems (Michael 2008).

It is essential you familiarise yourself with these associated health conditions and any potential health risks a person may be more vulnerable to or at increased risk of developing. This will enable you to spot any possible unmet health needs during assessments which may be affecting a person's functional performance during activities.

People who have a learning disability are likely to have difficulty recognising symptoms of an illness or health issue and may be unable to communicate them to carers and health professionals. Consequently there is a risk they will not receive diagnostic assessments, and necessary treatments, for health issues which may be present.

Sadly there have been cases where people with a learning disability have had health issues undetected, resulting in premature death. In such cases the health professional may have only considered the person's learning disability. This can result in *diagnostic overshadowing*, where the co-existing health needs of the person are not identified. *Death by Indifference* published by Mencap (2007), and the *Confidential Inquiry into Premature Deaths of People with Learning Disabilities* completed by Heslop *et al.* (2013) provide more information about this.

During occupational therapy assessments you may identify an unmet health need impacting on a person's functional performance. A referral may be required to other relevant health professionals for further assessment. Equally, the person may have health conditions which are detected but cannot be managed, resulting in them living with chronic pain, discomfort and sensory loss and so on. In such situations there may be a need for other health professionals to become involved, exploring effective ways to manage symptoms and optimise quality of life.

Changes in health and social care provision for people with learning disabilities

Before I describe current provision of services for people who have a learning disability I will provide you with an overview describing how these services have evolved over the years. This will help you understand the reasons behind practices and approaches used in occupational therapy today within learning disability teams.

The way in which people with a learning disability are supported and cared for within our society is very different from practice several decades ago. The National Learning Disabilities Professional Senate (2015) said that 'Life today is better for most individuals with Learning Disabilities and their families. However, there remain particular groups that remain at risk of unnecessary restrictive lifestyles, poor access to services and opportunities, and serious health inequalities.'

Over the last 20 years there have been media reports about how people with learning disabilities are supported and cared for in the community. Concerns regarding abuse and health inequalities have been highlighted, prompting inquiries, publication of white papers and legislation. The list below includes some of these reports and legislation influential in bringing about many of the changes in provision:

- *Valuing People* (Department of Health 2001)
- *Valuing People Now* (Department of Health 2009)
- *Learning Disability and Challenging Behaviour* (NICE guidelines) (National Institute of Clinical Excellence 2015)
- Mental Capacity Act 2005
- Autism Act 2009
- Equality Act 2010
- *Death by Indifference* (Mencap 2007) leading to *Healthcare for All* (Michael 2008)
- *Transforming Care* (Department of Health 2012) following on from the Winterbourne View inquiry
- *Confidential Inquiry into Premature Deaths of People with Learning Disabilities* (Heslop *et al.* 2013)

- *Delivering Effective Specialist Community Learning Disabilities Health Team Support to People with Learning Disabilities and Their Families or Carers* (National Learning Disabilities Professional Senate 2015).

Since the 1971 Department of Health white paper *Better Services for the Mentally Handicapped*, large institutions have closed, and teams have been formed to support people with a learning disability in the community; this situation was recognised in *Valuing People* (Department of Health 2001).

Concerns remained regarding how services were coordinated and planned, carer support, unmet healthcare needs, limited housing choice and employment opportunities, alongside a lack of person-centred day service provision, and individuals having little choice or control over many aspects of their lives.

Valuing People identified four key principles:

- rights
- independence
- choice
- inclusion.

The paper outlined how these principles could be implemented in practice. However, in 2007 *Death by Indifference* (Mencap 2007) highlighted continuing health inequalities within the population of people with learning disabilities, further identifying the need for improvements in health screenings, checks and reasonable adjustments, enabling people to access mainstream health services to meet their needs.

In response to *Death by Indifference* an inquiry into health services for people with learning disabilities was completed, leading to the publication of *Healthcare for All* (Michael 2008). The inquiry acknowledged this vulnerable group of people often have high health needs. Following this, a further inquiry, *Confidential Inquiry into Premature Deaths of People with Learning Disabilities* (Heslop *et al.* 2013) was completed.

It came to light that many people with a learning disability were unable to access some health services. Several reasons were identified, including limited knowledge of learning disability among general healthcare staff, lack of adjustments in relation to communication, cognitive impairment, choice and treatment preferences. Additionally, a need for collaboration with parents and carers, and improved communication between general health services and specialist learning disability teams was required.

The reports called for people with learning disabilities to be treated as equal citizens and to have equal access to healthcare treatment. It was, however, acknowledged that *equal* does not always mean *the same*, and that reasonable adjustments were needed to make services equitable for people with learning disabilities.

The Mental Capacity Act 2005 brings significant change in health and social care provision. This has been important in protecting rights of people with a learning disability and, as you will see, underpins many recommendations made in *Healthcare for All* (Michael 2008).

This legislation states adults with disabilities have the right to make their own decisions. To enable a person to make a decision information must be presented in a way people who have learning disabilities can understand, for example using easy read print, pictures and so on, or explaining in a different way.

If a decision is too complex for a person to make, all relevant people who care for them should be involved in making a 'best interest' decision on their behalf.

USEFUL WEB RESOURCE

www.mencap.org.uk/advice-and-support/mental-capacity-act

Unfortunately, even with these inquiries and legislation to improve the health and quality of life for those with learning disabilities, the abuse at Winterbourne View Hospital occurred. Following the exposure of this in 2011, a government report, *Transforming Care* (Department of Health 2012), was written. This document recommended a reduction in use of in-patient facilities, for people to live closer to families or familiar communities with the support needed, reduction of restrictive practices including the use of medication and a move towards positive behavioural support.

All of these inquiries, white papers and legislation shape how we work as occupational therapists with people who have a learning disability. If you are unfamiliar with the documents listed above, I recommend you study them; they will provide you with context of how services work and considerations for your own practice. I will refer to some of these documents as I talk more about the occupational therapist's role.

Consent and the Mental Capacity Act (MCA)

It is essential you have a good understanding of the MCA 2005. This act protects everyone's rights, including those of people who have a learning disability. In practice, this means you must identify if the person has mental capacity to consent to assessments and interventions you offer.

People who have a learning disability often find it difficult to understand and process new information. The way in which information is presented to them has a bearing on how much they understand and can retain. You will need to consider how you present information about assessments and interventions. This may involve talking to family and carers to decide the best method of communication. Information may need to be presented to the person using pictures, simplified written information, objects relating to the assessments or simple words.

If you identify a person who does not have the mental capacity to consent to any assessments or interventions, a *best interest* meeting and decision are required. This ensures all different considerations and opinions are heard, confirming proposed assessments and interventions are required and in the person's best interest.

Consent and any best interest decision should always be documented. It is worth noting consent has to be *specific* to the planned activity or intervention.

Service provision for people with learning disabilities

Having a learning disability affects all aspects of a person's life. The degree of learning disability and presence of associated physical, sensory needs and mental illness are likely to require involvement from primary and secondary health and social care teams, plus other 'care providing' agencies in the wider community. Generally, most social care teams are funded by county councils, with learning disability health teams funded by the NHS.

There is country-wide variation regarding how social care and NHS health teams are structured. Some social care teams have designated social workers and case coordinators working specifically with people who have learning disabilities and are separate from learning disability health teams. In other areas there are large generic social care teams working with all adults, including those people who have a learning disability. Alternatively, social care and NHS nursing teams are integrated, and allied health professions work in separate teams.

The difference in functions between social care and health teams is usually clearly defined. Generally, social care teams identify support people require to complete daily activities. A social worker completes a 'needs assessment'. There are occasions when the health team may need to contribute to this assessment in relation to the individual's health. If a person lives with their family, a 'carer's assessment' is completed.

How services are funded varies, and is dependent on individual need. There is a variety of funding streams; some care provision may be solely funded by social care or NHS, including Continuing Health Care (CHC), or a combination of both. The funding source impacts on the role of the care coordinator, who may, in some cases, be an occupational therapist.

CHC is NHS funded and provided when a person's primary need for care relates to their health. Some people who have a learning disability have complex physical health conditions and require care to meet health-related needs. In these situations the person's care is funded through CHC and the care coordinator within the learning disability team will be involved in regular reviews.

RECOMMENDED READING

The National Learning Disabilities Professional Senate paper (2015) provides a good description of the roles of each profession. Reading this before you start working in this clinical area ensures you have a good understanding of these different roles.

The role of the learning disabilities health team

The role of the learning disabilities health team is to identify and meet health needs affected by the person's learning disability.

The assessments and interventions provided are varied, complex and require a multi-disciplinary holistic approach. In many cases this also involves collaborative working with other healthcare teams, social care and care providers.

Occupational therapists working in a learning disabilities team are usually employed by the NHS within an MDT.

Health team members include:

- speech and language therapists (SALT)
- community learning disability nurses
- clinical psychologists
- physiotherapists
- consultant psychiatrists
- dieticians
- behavioural specialists.

I often think of the multi-disciplinary team as being like a machine, such as a car. The parts of the car: engine, wheels, steering, brakes and so on, can work in isolation but to make the car move or function they must work together. In the same way, different professionals can complete assessments, but to gain a holistic understanding of the person's needs and make an impact on their life, each assessment, intervention and recommendation must be viewed together to see the overall picture. If this does not happen, the isolated assessments and interventions could potentially be ineffective.

In most cases a person's identified needs impact on each other and are interconnected. Without communication strategies in place the person's preferences and choices cannot be identified in relation to preferred activities. Without postural support they cannot maintain a comfortable, functional position to participate in activity. Without meaningful activities a person is less likely to communicate, move, and utilise skills and abilities; ultimately this could lead to development of health problems. I hope this illustrates why collaborative multi-disciplinary team working is so essential in learning disabilities teams.

The occupational therapy role

There is often confusion amongst health professionals, including occupational therapists working in different settings, about what we actually do in learning disability teams.

The occupational therapy role is varied in learning disabilities, and I think this is a reflection of the needs of the population of people we work with. After all, people with learning disabilities are a diverse group of people, whose needs can vary hugely.

The complex needs of people with learning disabilities means there is a risk of trying to do everything and being 'Jack of all trades and master of none'. For this reason it is important to have a definition and clear understanding of the occupational therapy role, and how this differs from occupational therapists working in other settings.

If a person's occupational difficulties and needs primarily relate to a physical or mental illness, and not their learning disability, then it is important they access the specialist occupational therapy services those without learning disabilities access. This ensures they receive equitable and appropriate services to meet their health need as advocated in *Health for All* (Michael 2008). Part of our role is to support people accessing relevant mainstream services. At times this may involve you working collaboratively with occupational therapists in other settings.

Lillywhite and Haines (2010, p.1) describe the role of the occupational therapist in learning disabilities as:

> to maintain, restore, or create a beneficial match between an individual's abilities, the demands of their occupations and the demands of the environment, in order to maintain or improve their functional status and access to opportunities for participation. This can involve helping someone learn new ways of doing activities, adapting equipment or materials used every day and making changes to the places where they live and work.

Our role as occupational therapists in learning disabilities requires us to consider how an individual's learning disability impacts on their occupational performance, in other words, how their learning disability affects their engagement and performance in chosen activities.

A referral to a learning disability occupational therapist may be made for the following reasons:

- There are barriers preventing the person engaging in meaningful activities. These may be due to the physical environment, the approach and support provided during activities, sensory, mental health and/or physical disabilities a person may have.
- A person does not have opportunities to participate in a balance of occupations (self-care, work and leisure activities) and this has an impact on their physical and/or mental health.
- There are changes in a person's skills resulting in impact on their participation in chosen occupations.

Reports such as *Valuing People Now* (Department of Health 2009), the National Learning Disabilities Professional Senate paper (2015) and the *Learning Disabilities and Challenging Behaviour* guidelines (NICE 2015) highlight the importance of meaningful occupation for people with learning disabilities. The information provided in the *Transforming Care* document (Department of Health 2012) indicates that people lacked opportunities to engage in meaningful activities, and occupational deprivation is evident. In addition, evidence suggests people with learning disabilities are more likely to experience occupational deprivation and social isolation (Stancliffe *et al.* 2007).

The LD Senate paper (2015) advocates that participation in meaningful activities, such as self-care, work/domestic and leisure activities, could reduce the impact of mental illness, sensory and physical disabilities, challenging behaviours and social isolation. This in turn potentially reduces health inequalities and improves a person's quality of life.

Lillywhite and Haines (2010) advise occupational therapists in learning disabilities teams work with people in relation to physical and sensory disabilities, mental health diagnosis, dementia, autism, epilepsy and challenging behaviours. The skills and training we have makes us well placed to work in this area to identify and meet sensory and occupational needs.

To help describe the role in more detail, I have outlined assessments and interventions used within learning disabilities in three main areas:

- 'behaviours that challenge'

- profound and multiple learning disabilities (PMLD)
- dementia.

We also work with people with both a mental health condition and learning disability, and I provide a brief summary of what the occupational therapy role may entail.

Within all these areas there is overlap in the approaches, assessments and interventions used in practice.

Behaviours that challenge

According to *Learning Disability and Challenging Behaviour* (NICE 2015), people who have a learning disability sometimes display 'behaviours that challenge'. These behaviours can be self-injurious, aggressive towards other people and objects, show withdrawal, be disruptive or could result in involvement with the criminal justice system.

There may be a variety of reasons why a person may display 'behaviours that challenge'. NICE (2015) suggests they may be seeking sensory stimulation, attracting attention, avoiding demands and trying to communicate information with other people, such as feeling pain. When we talk about sensory stimulation, we mean tactile, vestibular, proprioceptive, auditory, visual, olfactory and gustatory stimulation.

The occupational opportunities available to a person, support they receive and physical and social environments can influence how a person feels, and contribute to displays of behaviours that challenge. This may be due to lack of social interaction, meaningful occupation, opportunity to make choices or stimulation to meet sensory needs, or due to excessive noise or unpredictable and unresponsive crowded environments.

NICE (2015) recommends performance skills and sensory assessments are completed and there are person-centred and meaningful activities available to the individual.

Initial assessments may need to be completed in collaboration with other team members to establish the risks of the person's behaviours, and if there are any underlying unmet health needs which should be addressed, for example a person may display a behaviour which is challenging because they are trying to communicate pain. There are a number of different models of practice which can be employed to promote holistic and client-centred practice. The Model of Human

Occupational Screening Tool (Parkinson, Forsyth and Kielhofner 2006) is a framework I can recommend.

Initial occupational therapy assessments may indicate further specific assessments are needed; these can relate to environmental barriers, such as the physical (e.g. light, temperature, furniture), social (e.g. noise, number of people, interactions), communication, complexity of an activity, range of activities and the relevance of occupations to the person.

All of these areas need to be considered and assessed. For example, if the person does not receive the type of support they require this may disempower them, leading to frustrations they are unable to communicate verbally, potentially leading to behaviours that challenge.

There are a range of other assessments, such as the Residential Environmental Impact Survey (REIS), Pool Activity Level (Pool 2008) and Sensory Processing Measure (SPM), which are useful in assessing a person's needs. These are only examples and others are available.

During the assessment process it may be identified that a person has unmet sensory needs and may have sensory processing difficulties. In this situation a specialist sensory integration (SI) assessment may be required. In simple terms, sensory integration is when the brain interprets information coming in from all the senses (tactile, vestibular, proprioceptive, auditory, visual, olfactory and gustatory) happening at a conscious and unconscious level. If there are issues with how this information is received and interpreted by the body and brain it can lead to difficulties adjusting and responding to sensations received (Goodman *et al.* 2009). If a person has SI difficulties, specialist assessments need to be undertaken by a clinician who has completed sensory integration training.

Occupational therapy interventions need to be carried out in collaboration with the client, carers/family and other professionals. Interventions involve providing information and education regarding activity grading to promote engagement in meaningful activities, adapting physical and social environments, increasing awareness of sensory processing difficulties and advising on meeting sensory needs.

Profound and multiple learning disabilities (PMLD)

People who have a PMLD will have more than one disability, their primary disability being a profound learning disability. They will have difficulty communicating and many will have additional sensory or physical disabilities, complex health needs or mental health difficulties. This group of people are dependent on others to understand and meet all their needs (Mansell 2010). These intellectual and physical disabilities mean there are more difficulties and barriers to overcome to access and engage in meaningful occupations. In *Raising Our Sights: Services for Adults with Profound Intellectual and Multiple Disabilities* (2010) Mansell advocates people with PMLDs need more support and opportunities to access and participate in meaningful activities.

Mansell then makes seven recommendations in relation to 'accessing buildings and communities', 'educational opportunities' and 'employment and leisure activities'. This document provides useful information about how to overcome some of the potential barriers and increase opportunities for people with PMLDs to access meaningful activities within their community.

Occupational deprivation is a great risk for people who have a PMLD. A person can suffer from lack of physical and mental stimulation, social isolation and lack of movement or change of position, all of which can have a detrimental effect on a person's physical and mental health. If a person is unable to communicate they will be understimulated or bored; this can lead them to displaying behaviours that challenge.

Occupational therapists have an important role to support and implement the recommendations made in *Raising Our Sights*. Kielhofner (2008) describes how we can complete holistic assessments enabling us to identify the person's cognitive and physical skills, and environmental barriers impacting on the person's performance and engagement in daily activities. Occupational therapists have knowledge and skills in activity analysis, activity grading and adaptation of the environment and tasks. These skills enable them to develop goals and interventions with individuals, promoting optimum participation in occupations with meaning to the person.

People who have a PMLD are likely to have skills at an early stage of development, this means they may engage in activities at a sensory level. In other words, the person interacts and engages in the activity through the sensory experience whether it is tactile, vestibular, proprioceptive, auditory, visual, olfactory or gustatory.

During the assessment stage it is important to establish if the person has sensory impairments, their sensory preferences and if there are indications to suggest they may have any sensory integration issues. If these are indicated further assessments by a specialist sensory integration occupational therapist may be needed. Part of the assessment and work may also involve collaboration with adult social care occupational therapists to address physical environmental barriers restricting a person participating in an activity.

It is also likely speech and language therapists (SALT) and physiotherapists will work alongside occupational therapists when developing goals and interventions to promote activity engagement with a person who has a PMLD. The person's communication is likely to be limited; support from the speech and language therapists to identify strategies to enhance their interaction, choice making and engagement will be required.

Awareness of the person's posture and functional position when they participate in an activity may require joint working with physiotherapy. Equally, it may be the physiotherapist who is working with the individual to maintain posture, and an occupational therapy assessment is required to identify meaningful activities they can engage in to support this work.

A person who has a PMLD will be more dependent on carers and family to provide occupational opportunities and support to engage in activity. It is vital you work closely with carers and families when completing assessments and planning interventions.

It is easy to forget how your knowledge and skills were developed in relation to adapting activities supporting engagement and participation in an activity. It is important not to assume that families and carers will be able to take information and recommendations made in reports and transfer them into real-life situations when supporting a person to engage in an activity. It may be necessary to provide training sessions, modelling and use of technology such as films to provide support and ongoing information.

Dementia

People who have a learning disability are thought to be at greater risk of developing dementia than the general population (Cooper and van der Speck 2009). According to the Alzheimer's Society approximately 1 in 5 people with a learning disability over the age of 65 will develop dementia. It is also estimated that 1 in 50 people with Down's syndrome develop dementia in their 30s, rising sharply to more than half of those who live to 60 or over (Alzheimer's Society 2017).

Occupational therapists contribute to the assessment information required for the accurate diagnosis of dementia. According to Kottorp

(2008), the AMPS can be used to provide a measure of a person's motor and process skills. This assessment can be repeated, alongside other psychological assessment, after a six-month period, to track changes and decline in a person's skills. This information provides a measure of change and can promote accuracy in diagnosis.

The need for occupational therapist does not cease once a dementia diagnosis is made, ongoing involvement is required. Nygard *et al.* (1994) suggest that the aim of occupational therapy for people with dementia is to maintain the person's functional performance and participation in activities. To achieve this an assessment of the person's level of skill is required. The information from AMPS can be used alongside additional assessments. The Pool Activity Level (Pool 2008) and REIS are useful tools. Information gained from these assessments enables occupational therapists to develop goals with individuals and carers, making recommendations in relation to adapting activities and physical environments and supporting the promotion of engagement and participation in activities. This will require ongoing support from carers and family.

At some point this work may involve working with occupational therapists in other areas, such as social care. It is likely the person's physical abilities will change in the longer term. Assessments may indicate the home environment meets the person's current needs but, in time, as skills change, physical adaptations and/or equipment may be required to maintain participation in activities for as long as possible. It is beneficial to introduce any equipment or changes as early as possible. This will enable the individual to familiarise themselves with these changes whilst cognitive ability to adapt remains.

A referral can be made to occupational therapists working in social care teams for assessments and interventions. It is good practice to work jointly in these situations, so holistic assessments in relation to the person's learning disability and physical environmental needs are considered. It is also a great opportunity for CPD, working with another therapist who has differing skills to yourself.

Mental health disorder/illness

People who have a learning disability are also vulnerable to developing mental illness. Research shows mental illness has a higher prevalence in the learning disability population in comparison to the general population (Cooper *et al.* 2007; Hardy, Chaplin and Woodward 2007).

Your role when working with people who have a learning disability and mental illness may require you to work collaboratively with mental health services. This may require supporting and advising mental health services to make 'reasonable adjustments' in relation to how information is provided, how assessments are introduced and carried out. In some situations the nature of the mental illness may not lead to the person accessing mainstream mental health services. Assessments and interventions will therefore need to be identified and used to understand how their learning disability and mental illness affects their participation in activities.

It is good practice to liaise with occupational therapists working in specialist areas, such as mental health teams, as these occupational therapists will be able to share information and skills which enable you to work effectively meeting the person's needs.

Not all people are the same!

There may be times when a referral will come into the learning disability team where a person presents with a particular diagnosis and clinical need, but how need is assessed and addressed may vary. Everybody is an individual, and their needs are individual. The most important thing is to identify what their health need is and the impact of their learning disability on health and quality of life.

Conclusion

I hope the information in this chapter has provided you with insight into being an occupational therapist in a learning disabilities team; there is so much to cover and only a small amount has been included in this chapter. The references used provide more in-depth information about specific areas and I strongly recommend you read them.

Working as an occupational therapist with people who have learning disabilities continues to give me a great deal of pleasure and satisfaction. I still experience a 'buzz' when the person I am working with, and the care team supporting them, achieve their goals and have a positive impact on their health and quality of life.

This clinical setting will provide you with lots of opportunities to work with a variety of people, with different professions and agencies.

Enjoy the diversity, and most of all enjoy what you do!

8

CHILDREN WITH DISABILITIES (SOCIAL CARE)

Ruth Parker

Introduction

Congratulations, you have decided that working with children with disabilities (CWD) is for you!

First, minimising confusion, I use 'CWD' to differentiate between community paediatric occupational therapists and teams based within social care. There are areas of overlap and, indeed, some teams are integrated. (If you apply for a job and are not 100 per cent sure of the team's role or remit – ask! This is an instance when asking a 'stupid' question (a) prevents embarrassment at interview, and (b) ensures you don't waste time gathering in-depth information in areas not required.) If you are applying to, or joining, an integrated team, reading this chapter in conjunction with the paediatrics chapter is recommended.

So, you are joining the world of social care working with children with disabilties; what exactly does this mean? Generally, you are employed by a local authority (LA) with responsibility to provide support for children and young people (YP) with disabilities in their home environment. This responsibility is detailed in Section 17 (10) of the Children Act 1989, to safeguard and promote the interests of 'children in need', this description is recognised in law as including children with disabilities.

Here, for the most part, we leave the medical model behind, viewing the world through the lens of the social model of disability. As a result, we do not have 'patients', but children, YP, parents, carers, families...often referred to by a 'catch all' term such as 'service user'. Whilst occupational therapists working in social care work within the social model of disability, our understanding of medical conditions and the medical model supports interventions and clinical reasoning. This holistic approach is important as we complete casework and support families.

If you envisage your role as one where you spend time assessing children's development and engaging in therapeutic play activities, I am afraid you need to think again (unless you are joining an integrated team, or have just realised you are reading the wrong chapter!).

Our role seeks to maximise children's and young people's abilities, supporting caregiving in the home environment, considering aspects including stage of development, cognition and awareness of safety. Equally important is the family/care structure around children. Whilst our focus places children at the centre of attention, they cannot be seen in a vacuum. They are surrounded by family, carers and others, and in an environment affecting their, and others', ability to participate in occupations.

Continuing in this chapter I use the term 'child' – what I mean is anyone up to the age of 18 (or whichever age is used as the upper age in a team's criteria).

Stages of development and conditions

A quick dip back in to the medical model now, as our knowledge of typical child development and understanding of medical conditions provide foundations on which we base clinical reasoning and recommendations.

'Age and stage' is a phrase some use as a benchmark against which findings are considered following an assessment, but this cannot be a hard and fast rule. It remains age appropriate for a toddler to wear nappies and for the majority of their needs to be met by others. Our skill is to understand how conditions/diagnoses alter over subsequent years, enabling us to promote independence, occupations and facilitate care. If a toddler has a condition you know will deteriorate, this must be taken into consideration but is not the sole, nor main, area of attention. This knowledge and understanding is one piece of a jigsaw you construct through your time working with the child and their family.

There will be conditions recorded as a diagnosis seen frequently, such as cerebral palsy (CP) or muscular dystrophy (MD). There will also be many you will only come across once or twice, or even those without a name (often referred to as 'syndrome without a name' or SWAN). Remember that each of these is only a label, in every instance the child and family's experience is different. Indeed, terms such as cerebral palsy or muscular dystrophy are just classifications, within these symptoms and progression differs. The progression of Duchenne muscular dystrophy is different to myotonic or distal muscular dystrophy, and cerebral palsy may be classified by severity level, parts of the body affected, the extent of impact on motor function and so on. There aren't enough words in this book to cover even the most common conditions you will find and this isn't the remit of this chapter.

There are useful resources in this chapter and most named conditions have a society or support group with a web presence. These not only outline conditions but often include information on difficulties children and their families encounter. A word of caution – whilst this may be useful, you are assessing the situation a child and their family are *actually* experiencing. This where your abilities to assess, analyse activities and to clinically reason are key to ensuring actions you propose and outcomes you aim for are appropriate. There is no point in working on a presumption a child with Duchenne muscular dystrophy is a wheelchair user by the age of 11, if the 11-year-old in front of you remains mobile. In these situations you seek to meet identified needs but with an eye on meeting future needs, using your knowledge with guidance from multi-disciplinary team members considering long-term prognosis.

Not all children have physical needs, some result from challenging behaviours, some a combination of both. This is a relatively new area of intervention for many teams and often there is lack of wider support, with intervention services limited. Considerations when assessing the impact of challenging behaviours include safety of the child and of others in a household. The underlying cause may not be apparent but may be linked to diagnosis, sensory issues, communication difficulties or frustration. In some situations equipment or adaptation may be indicated, these should follow work with both child and parents addressing problem behaviours; equipment/adaptation is generally a last resort. This is not always possible; your knowledge of local interventions and support ensures your recommendations are appropriate and timely.

> If considering equipment or adaptations to assist with managing challenging behaviour, remember how these can potentially be used. There may be issues with deprivation of liberty or restraint which need to be considered alongside your assessment of hazards and risks.

Team

You are not alone in this new world. Teams not only support families but also their members. This wider team is like a jigsaw – but one where not all pieces are needed at one time to complete the picture!

The structure of any team supporting a child depends on their and their family's needs and services offered within an area. Within social care you will work with social workers (SW), but not every child requires SW support; other members of this wider team may include sensory support staff, Early Help, health visitors and *education, health and care* (EHC) plan caseworkers.

There will be links with paediatric occupational therapists, speech and language therapists and physiotherapists. As early interventions are usually within a child's home this is where boundaries can become blurred and good communication key – joint working opportunities are encouraged! There may be an agreement in place to clarify roles, or it may be on a case-by-case basis. The key is to understand structures in your area, this supports joint working and minimises confusion for families.

Others in the multi-disciplinary team with whom you will have close working relationships are those in working in housing and adaptations. Once again, areas differ in approach. Some councils have occupational therapists working within housing departments; all will have housing officers, but they may have a different title. Social housing needs may be met 'in house' or may have been devolved to social landlords/housing associations, adaptations may be via Disabled Facilities Grant (DFG) process or separate funding. If a local authority area covers a number of different councils (city, borough or district), it is likely each will have different methods for applications and for what they will consider funding. Chapter 10, 'Adaptations', will help towards your understanding, but building local knowledge is essential.

There is a team around the child but there is also one around you! You may be co-located with occupational therapists or be the sole occupational therapist within a team of social workers. If you are lucky enough to be with occupational therapists, they will have a wealth of knowledge, but remember social workers will have worked with families receiving occupational therapy support; they too will be able to offer you advice and information on aspects of your work.

One last thought on team working. Your decision-making and recommendations are not made in isolation. An example: recommending a stair lift for a child whose physio outcome is to improve stair climbing ability is counter-productive – liaison is key!

Voice of the child (VOC) and communicating with children with disabilities

Hearing and recording the voice of the child is a key theme across all aspects of paediatrics. Where a child is without cognitive impairment and able to articulate thoughts and opinions this is relatively easy. 'Relatively', as children may articulate what they *think* the listener wishes to hear or what they consider to be in line with their parent's wishes. As your involvement may continue for months or years, revisiting conversations to see if a child's opinions or thoughts have altered is good practice.

You will, of necessity, in many cases, rely on parents and carers to explain a child's needs and preferences. It is, however, essential to include and evidence the VOC in both your assessment and decision-making. For children who do not use verbal communication you will need to develop an understanding of methods they may use to communicate. These include British Sign Language (BSL), Makaton, Picture Exchange Communication System (PECS) or objects of reference or assistive technology. You do not need to be proficient in all of these but if your information gathering identifies a communication method it should be (a) recorded and (b) used to communicate with the child wherever possible.

Communication is a two-way street; where a child has a visual or hearing impairment, consideration of how you share information or discuss issues is required. We cannot all be fluent in BSL or Makaton but there will be ways to communicate. Liaising with parents and school or local support services may assist in identifying the most appropriate methods – use the members of the multi-disciplinary team to support your work.

Children who are non-verbal, or who do not interact with you, present challenges when recording their thoughts and opinions. Your first consideration should be 'Is it realistic to elicit a response?' Asking a child with a cognitive impairment their thoughts in regard to architectural plans is unrealistic but asking them (through image, symbol, etc.) if they prefer a shower or bath informs understanding and decision-making. When trying equipment or introducing a new method of completing a task, observation of facial expression and body language enables your records to show how a child felt about a particular intervention.

This is not to say that recording the VOC is always difficult. Seeing a child complete an activity or achieve a personal aim may result in laughter, tears, smiles and so on and recording that 'child X completed the activity unaided, and on completion smiled and bounced up and down with excitement' is a clear indication of their feelings. For a teenager, a nod of the head and 'it's OK' may be the highest praise you can expect.

A child's voice need not necessarily be heard only through vocalisation; they may be able to draw a picture indicating preferences or feelings. If there is opportunity during a visit then this may be a chance to work directly with a child but, if not, why not suggest they could draw something for you later?

Children are just that, children, so do remember they have good days and bad days and you will meet the 'terrible twos' and sulky teenagers. A child may not be enthused by the prospect of adaptations to support personal care activities – engagement may not be forthcoming when discussing toileting, not a hot topic but essential. Don't forget the impact of embarrassment as well.

Many visits follow a school day, possibly after a long journey home (many children with disabilities attend school some distance from home) so perfect behaviour cannot really be expected. In fact, seeing a child on an 'off day' may provide more insight than when they are at their best, although parents are often embarrassed and require reassurance that the occupational therapist understands and is not judgemental.

Assessment

Assessment is the foundation underpinning occupational therapy interventions and working with children with disabilities is no different. Whilst diagnosis of a child's condition provides you with an idea of what their abilities and prognosis may be, each and every situation is different.

Information gathering is key to understanding the support network around the child. Working in a child's home means taking into consideration the family unit. An unfortunate fact is the higher than average number of children with disabilities who live in single parent family units. Understanding what, or if any, support is offered by the absent parent should always be recorded, as this aids your understanding of their situation. Children may also be in the care of members of the wider family (grandparents, aunts, siblings) or be fostered, either privately or in the care of the local authority. Understanding who has parental responsibility assists in identifying who should be consulted or involved with decision-making. Within this network of support you will also need to find out about school or nursery (mainstream/special school), home-based support (portage, domiciliary care, etc.), involved therapists and children's leisure activities.

Families come in many shapes and sizes, the roles and abilities of all members require consideration. Parents may have their own health issues and, where a child requires a high level of support for transfers, or care support is given in a less than ideal situation, musculoskeletal injuries are all too often an issue. Treatment for these is complicated by necessity to continue to meet care needs, meaning the cause of an injury cannot be avoided.

Siblings too may have health issues or disabilities which may require an assessment to identify their needs. Even if this is not the case, they should always be considered. Recommendations made impact on all family members and, while you may not be able to minimise this, acknowledging their impact may make them more acceptable. Siblings of a children with disabilities may also assist with caregiving, therefore understanding and recognising this support is essential. If this is the case, signposting to services to support young carers may be an option (but remember to obtain consent before making a referral).

Safeguarding

This is a concern for children with disabilities as much as for any group of children. Families with a child with a disability may have increased stress and are often more isolated. The National Society for the Prevention of Cruelty to Children (NSPCC) advise this group are in fact at greater risk than non-disabled peers (NSPCC 2016). Children without communication difficulties find this a difficult subject to discuss, this can only be increased for a child who (a) cannot communicate and (b) may be reliant on their abuser for personal care or access to activities. This area also includes radicalisation and domestic abuse; focus should not be limited to the child we are assessing but all family members. There will be training offered by your employer/organisation but wider reading is recommended to assist in understanding the signs indicating abuse, different types of abuse and, most importantly, the correct actions when abuse is suspected.

Knowledge

You will have graduated with a head full of 'stuff' – some of it very interesting but not immediately relevant in your new role. I can't tell you what you will need to know, but can point you in the right direction and advise you will never stop learning.

Chapter 12 on legislation will be a good place to start. The remit of the children with disabilities occupational therapist's role is linked to the Chronically Sick and Disabled Persons Act 1970 and Children and Families Act 2014. For children transitioning to adulthood the Care Act 2014 applies. It will also be essential to have a working knowledge of the Mental Capacity Act 2005 for your work with older children.

One area requiring thorough knowledge is the Housing Grants, Construction and Regeneration Act 1996. This provides criteria for eligibility and which adaptations can be provided via this funding stream (see Chapters 10 and 12).

There will be mandatory training in areas such as manual handling, domestic abuse, radicalisation and safeguarding. These may be delivered as e-learning packages or face-to-face training. Your awareness supports you in your work, alongside social work colleagues, in identifying signs and considering appropriate actions if you have areas of concern.

Equipment and adaptations

Appearances may be deceptive, education and therapeutic interventions may appear to be key activities in a child's life but, remember this, a child spends more time at home than in other settings.

Interventions in the home support a child getting up, accessing bathing and toileting, eating, getting out of the house to go to school, play, sleep... You get the gist?

Supporting these essential occupations enables children to go to school, reduces stress linked to caregiving activities and therefore supports a positive start and end to the day. Our role enables us to set up firm foundations for children with disabilities and their parents, facilitating independence and care in the home environment. It may appear as 'quiet' work completed in the background of a child's life but is an essential support.

Equipment

Equipment provision supporting occupations in the home is an ongoing process. As children grow needs alter as skills are mastered or, for those with degenerative conditions, additional support is required to compensate.

There is a wide range of equipment available and attendance at trade shows such as Naidex or Kidz may leave you reeling at choice, colours or just at names of items. No longer will you talk about 'shower chairs' or 'seating' – welcome to a world of Seahorses, Flamingos, Tritons and Bees!

Bringing it back to basics, equipment choices are pretty much the same as for adults, supporting occupations such as bathing, toileting, showering and so on. The greatest difference is found in seating/postural management and in bed provision. In some teams 24-hour postural management will be provided by occupational therapists, in others responsibility may be divided, with physiotherapists providing sleep systems and occupational therapists seating systems. Either way you will need to understand the principles of 24-hour postural management, measurement and prescription of equipment.

Seating systems promote occupations through provision of appropriate, comfortable support. There are systems designed primarily to provide supportive, comfortable seating; more commonly seating is prescribed to support occupations. These include personal care, feeding and homework but the most important occupation for children is play. Not play as therapy – play. Prescribed equipment may support therapeutic interventions based around playful activities but this is not the key consideration.

A slight digression on a subject close to my heart – play. Paraphrasing a number of definitions:

> Play is an occupation children engage in which is freely experienced, with no other purpose than enjoyment.

All too often for children with disabilities 'play' activities are linked to learning and mastering a skill. There is nothing intrinsically wrong with this. Play for children without impairments can be a learning tool but they also have opportunities 'just' to play. Asking a child or their carers what play activities they enjoy and how these are facilitated may highlight an area of need missed in discussions around personal care needs. The complexity of meeting care needs may mean this key occupation becomes less of a focus. Provision of sensory toys enjoyed whilst lying on the floor is most probably not within your team's remit; facilitating the transfer from seating to floor most certainly is!

Off my soapbox and on with the topic.

Profiling or 'hospital' beds are often prescribed for adults; however, for children with disabilities there are additional considerations. A child's size may mean risk of entrapment is greater and limited awareness of risk or danger requires particular care when prescribing mattresses and bed safety (cot) sides. Conversely, for a bed for a child without cognitive impairment, of an adult size, an 'adult' specification may be suitable.

Where a profiling bed is not appropriate provision a cot bed may be required. These adult-size beds have sides of varying heights and can have padding, clear Perspex panels and/or spindles. Cot beds are often bespoke, adapted to the needs of an individual child. As with any equipment prescribed, clinical reasoning and risk assessment evidences requirement for something which may at first seem an extreme solution.

Things to consider when assessing for a bed or cot bed: first, provision will usually be for long-term need – will a teenager still appreciate the colour scheme chosen when they were six? A shorter length cot bed may appear 'appropriate' for a toddler but not suitable when they mature into a lanky teenager. This is not to say all beds should be beige and boring, neither should they lead to future requests as appearance or length are no longer age appropriate. Second, how flexible is the bed or cot bed in meeting changing abilities? The assessment and provision process can be intrusive and adapting to new equipment unsettling. Third, why is the bed required? If it is to meet medical need then it may be more appropriate for a nurse to prescribe. Prescribers attempt to cover as many variables as possible, often within tight timescales, so will not always get it right, but looking at as many facets of need as possible should cover most situations.

Not all equipment is issued to facilitate needs of a child. Carers, informal (family members) or formal (domiciliary care workers), are considered within occupational therapy assessments. Where assistance with personal care is required it should be completed in an appropriate location, considering the dignity and safety of both the child receiving care and the carer.

Prescription is not the end of the story; children grow, needs and abilities alter, equipment is reviewed, adjusted or replaced. Teams have their own processes for reviewing equipment but advising parents to step back and look at how well their child is supported by, or fits in, their equipment prepares them for the reassessment process. Some parents are proactive, whilst others wait for scheduled reviews. Good practice at the point of prescription is ensuring parents are aware of processes for reporting faults or repairs but also how to request reassessment. Decision-making around equipment for younger children will often rely heavily on parents but always, where possible, involve the child. This in time supports not only good practice but also obligations under the MCA 2005 for those over 16.

A slight aside linked to equipment provision. Each team has access to 'stock' equipment from a central store either run in-house or outsourced. Considering stock items is *always* your first step in the assessment and prescription process. If no suitable option is identified, then a non-contract item is your next option. Generally, there will be non-contract items returned to stores, serviced and refurbished for reissue. Considering if these meet identified need is the next step. After this you will need to look at alternative options. This may mean asking team members for support or requesting a demonstration by a company rep. Whilst reps are very knowledgeable their role is *secondary* to your assessment, clinical reasoning and decision-making.

When relatively inexperienced, it is reassuring to have someone supporting you but it is important to maintain a balance. It is your responsibility to make final decisions on what should or should not be prescribed. If decisions are challenged, you will have evidence supporting your decision-making. Support, information and advice from peers will help you build up knowledge and confidence, so make use of your colleagues as much as you can.

> The Disabled Living Foundation (DLF) has fact sheets and independent information covering a range of paediatric equipment – useful for both occupational therapists and parents.

The wide range of equipment available may lead to situations where parental preference differs from your recommendation. This can lead to conflict but as long as your clinical reasoning is clear and recorded the evidence is in place to support your position. Clarity of advice and information from the start assists in managing expectations.

Parents' caring roles may extend beyond an age where usually a child becomes independent. At times approaches to caregiving may not alter to reflect growing maturity. If this is the case tact and diplomacy are required when discussing this. Whilst changing a baby's nappy wherever is most convenient is a choice many parents make, continuing this practice for a maturing child should be questioned, not only to maintain dignity but also to reduce the impact of caregiving in a less than ideal situation. It may not be possible to alter practice but, unless this is highlighted, parents' focus on meeting care needs may override reflection on how they complete these tasks.

Increasingly medical interventions and support available to children with complex conditions result in extended life expectancy. Also, where previously children with disabilities could not be supported outside a hospital environment, they are supported at home by family and carers. This presents challenges; assessing need for a child requiring complex medical support, whose progress cannot be predicted, will require joint multi-disciplinary team working.

Experience, our own and others' (multi-disciplinary team, clinicians, parents and carers, etc.) combines, providing a general understanding of how a child may progress. This supports our work with children with muscular dystrophy, Rett syndrome, cerebral palsy and other diagnoses we see frequently. Where we step into unknown territory we do not have references and experience to draw upon. Then it may well be our interventions are reactive to changes rather than planned, we may 'overprescribe' where a child's development exceeds expectation or find ourselves reassessing more frequently than predicted.

This serves to remind us every child's situation is unique, and our holistic approach to assessment must consider the individual, drawing on our experience and knowledge, alongside that of others, to inform our clinical reasoning, underpinning advice and information given, prescription of equipment, and recommendations for adaptations.

Adaptations

Adaptations are covered in more depth in Chapter 10, but children with disabilities is an area of practice where you cover the whole range. There will be occasions where a second stair rail, grab rail or threshold ramp meet need facilitating independence or identified need requires a ground floor bathroom and bedroom. Adaptations for children are not currently means tested but adaptations frequently exceed maximum grant allowances. As with equipment, our role is to consider both need and impact of provision…and to manage expectations.

Online information about the Disabled Facilities Grant may lead to expectation that the full grant limit (£30,000 in 2018) is available, resulting in parents planning 'their' adaptation prior to assessment of need, let alone completion of a recommendation. My advice? First read the relevant chapter in this book and, second, ensure you fully understand the grant process and criteria.

One area of confusion may be the amount awarded – the phrase 'up to' may not fully register. Families may feel short-changed when assessed need identifies the appropriate adaptation at a lower cost. Another area where a family's expectations may not correspond with (a) assessed need and (b) grant criteria may be the need to consider adaptation opportunities *within the scope of the current layout.* Our homes are close to our hearts and it may be difficult to accept a playroom or study could be utilised as a bedroom. Storage, or space for a carer to sleep in a bedroom, may also lead to discussions or disappointment. These are not within current grant criteria but equipment, incontinence pads and medications can overwhelm every nook and cranny in a home. You may also encounter resistance where family are reluctant to consider a child sleeping on a different level. Working through and around these points will be an important part of your role, liaising and mediating, until agreement can be found.

Each council or authority has their own processes by which adaptations are accessed. Increasingly for those requiring social housing, initial responses to requests for adaptation will be for families to consider rehousing to a more suitable property. Not an easy decision for many families and one where occupational therapists are an invaluable support in identifying the right property.

Manual handling

Transferring between equipment and rooms and so on is relatively simple when a child is young. As they grow and mature this need may possibly reduce as abilities increase; support is then via advice and information facilitating independent transfers. Where this is not possible, identifying appropriate methods is required, introducing these with sensitivity and tact. Some families embrace assisted transfers with hoists or other equipment, whilst others find this difficult. This may be linked to a belief they can 'manage', not appreciating the negative impact of long-term manual handling. Observing change when you are close to it is difficult; how often do parents suddenly realise how much a child has grown and new clothes are required? Parents know children grow but find themselves surprised year in year out. It may be that information and advice are enough to support the introduction of transfer equipment into the home. But reluctance to consider transfer equipment may link to difficulty in accepting a child's diagnosis or deterioration in their condition.

Conclusion

I hope this chapter has not left you feeling daunted, rather you are looking forward to taking on a role where days will be varied and interesting. Working with CWD is enjoyable, fun, frustrating, challenging. You will be in a position where you can make a positive difference to children's and parents' lives. At the end of a day, or at the end of casework, you will, in most cases, be able to reflect positively on your role. You will develop knowledge and experience across a wide range of interventions, which, if you feel the need to experience a different area of occupational therapy (although I can't see why you would want to!), will give you easily transferable skills.

Reflections

Parents of a child with a disability will have a grief or acceptance process they will go through. Some find an ability to adjust expectations after a relatively short time, whilst others may never fully accept their situation. This is not a linear process, and is dependent on stresses and strains in life and other factors. Proposing introduction of items of equipment at any time will require acceptance by both the child and their wider family. This can be most difficult when a need to consider hoisting is required. Seating, toileting and bathing equipment support other activities. The introduction of hoisting replaces assisted transfers and can be the step parents find most difficult.

I would like to add a couple of personal reflections. Where a child requires 24-hour postural support, the only time they are held by their parent may be during transfers. Removing this opportunity for 'hugs' or close contact should be considered a major change, which, whilst required to minimise risk, is a huge change for child and parent. Also, consider families where a child has developed along 'normal' patterns who then must adjust to a new reality. This may follow diagnosis of a condition, result from injury or illness or after treatment such as chemotherapy. These families often have to adjust to change in a very short timescale and a requirement to introduce complex equipment and hoist transfers is a huge adjustment.

Our role is to work with families and children, supporting them, enabling them to focus on family life and, as far as possible, minimising the impact of the child's disability. The ability to balance how and when an intervention is introduced is a skill refined as experience is gained. As a profession we have the ability to identify need and support positive changes through our interventions.

9

ADULT SOCIAL CARE

Julia Badger and Dawn Simm

Introduction

Hello and welcome to the ever-changing world of adult social care (ASC). If you are looking for a static role in occupational therapy, one where you can kick back and relax a bit, watch the world roll by as you gently absorb the ways of working, like a slow-cook risotto just bubbling on the surface, think again. ASC may not appear as fast-paced as an acute setting but demands are just as high.

You will not be working in a clinical setting with the environmental reassurances this can provide. You will work in the community, invariably in someone's home environment, with all the complexities and connotations attached to the meaning of the word 'home'. With this in mind, entering the world of ASC it may be beneficial for newly qualified occupational therapists with limited work/life experience to spend time in a more supported setting where they can expand their work/life skills. This way, they gain a deeper understanding of conditions and how these and co-morbidities impact upon function.

But please do not let that put you off! The role is extraordinarily rewarding and provides opportunities for you to use your hard-learned skills to support and invest in people, enabling them to make positive changes and optimise functional ability for the long term. If this has caught your attention then please read on, you will not be disappointed.

Working for ASC, it is more than likely you will be employed by a local authority in a multi-disciplinary team with social workers, support workers and business support (administration). Standard areas of work relate to long-term need and will include assessing need, service provision, reviewing services, manual handling and aids and adaptations (minor and major). Some adult social care teams are integrated with healthcare and provide rehabilitation/reablement, (short-term) interventions to promote independent living following a period of ill-health or following hospital discharge.

If you decide to apply for a job with adult social care, read the occupational therapist's job specification; ask what the role entails and how the team is set up before sending in the application form. Every job advertised has a small paragraph usually saying: 'For more information' or 'For an informal discussion contact...' *Do it, make the call.* There are no 'stupid' questions, you are information gathering, preparing for the task ahead – all basic occupational therapy skills. (Remember the Conscious Competence Learning Model?!) Understanding the role enables you to adapt your application, give examples of where you meet the job specifications, highlight your unique selling point and make yourself stand out from the occupational therapy crowd.

Integrating health and social care may appear disjointed but in fact is often the obvious way forward in the current political climate with its emphasis on budget control and cutbacks and is one of the aims of the Care Act 2014. Demands on services have increased and resources, that is, the people delivering the service, have been reduced. Health and social care overlap in many areas of service provision. The problem with this is gaps can appear; we may assume someone else will be providing a particular service. Thus people who need care and support can 'slip through the net'. It is far more productive for services to 'dovetail' and create a seamless service with clear pathways for those we work with to transition between. Good communication between services is vital and never assume...!

Equally, with collaborative working, any difficulties moving from a medical model to a social model of disability can be smoothed out, for example in identifying what is a short- or long-term intervention. Conflict and confusion can be reduced by making this transparent to the people using our services when they make the transition from hospital to return home.

Remember, a hospital is not a place to 'get well'; it is where we receive specialist medical treatment. If you have ever had to stay overnight or longer in a hospital you will know it is not a restful place. It is a busy alien environment, shared with people not of your choosing, where routines are restrictive. Home is usually the best place to 'get well' following specialist treatment in hospital. You are in a familiar environment, sights, sounds and smells. You can take back ownership of your daily routines. However, if your needs have significantly changed and you are unable to safely and independently access those essential activities of daily living, you may need long-term support, or aids or adaptations to enable you to remain at home. This is where the ASC occupational therapist steps up. They complete an assessment of need with you and plan interventions to support with role change and/or adapt the environment to promote safe, accessible, independent living.

Home

Take a few moments to consider what home means to you: the fact is, we complete some of our most personal and meaningful activities in the environment we call home. There could be positive or negative attachments. For some it is a refuge from the daily rigours and trials of life, a place to feel safe, our rock in a storm. For others, not so.

Memories can be attached to each area or item; whether you live alone or with family/others. Furniture is arranged in a way you feel suits your needs best. Everything you need may be around you within easy reach. Each article is significant and/or representative of your life and memories, your hard work and money are invested in this space.

> Write it all down. If you had to leave 'home' what would you want to take with you? What or who is important to you? Which activities or areas in your home would you be able to tolerate not having/doing without for a period of time? Think about how you would feel if another person, a stranger, steps into your life and 'home', making suggestions on how to make changes to improve your functional ability and quality of life within your living space.

Some people can accept change with open arms, others may be more reticent. Downsizing in later life can have significant impact on someone's feelings of self-worth, others may see it as freedom providing time to spend on leisure. It is essential you consider the dynamics of relationships within the home as this also influences an individual's ability to function and proactively engage in activities and/or interventions. Equally, consider the impact of loneliness, which will be discussed further later.

Adult social care team

The role of the adult social care team is to provide information, advice and/or support for individuals with an assessed physical or mental impairment or illness. The core driver behind this role is the Care Act 2014 and the statutory framework within the legislation incorporating:

- assessment
- eligibility
- care and support of assessed needs
- care and support guidance
- personalisation
- the wellbeing principle
- prevention.

The role can vary between local authorities but, by and large, it covers all adults from the age of 18. So this could be young people transitioning from children's services to adult mental health, learning disabilities and/or difficulties, older people, physical disabilities, end of life and so on.

We hope now you can understand why we suggest it is in your best interest to have good working/life knowledge and skills in all these areas.

The multi-disciplinary team will invariably include social workers, unqualified support workers and business support. If you are in an integrated team it may also include physiotherapists, nurses, rehabilitation support workers and so on. Use your induction period wisely and get to know the roles and responsibilities of your team colleagues. This will enable you to understand where you (and they) sit within the team and to work collaboratively to offer a seamless service.

Depending on where you are working geographically, you may find yourself in a small 'area' team or in a larger 'central' team. Get to know what services are available within your area, network with teams in other areas and share information. Get to know local health teams, snap up opportunities to 'shadow' or complete joint visits with your colleagues; it will give you a good understanding into their practice and the parameters they work within. Write everything down so you can refer back to names, contact details, role and so on – there will be a lot of information coming your way.

The word 'ever-changing' was used at the start of this chapter. It was not added glibly. The one constant in adult social care is that it will change. As politics evolves, with its efforts to improve public services, the influence on resources and ways of working will reverberate like ripples on a pond. Remember! You are working for a local authority and utilising public funding.

When you have worked in social care for a period of time and a 'new' system is introduced you will find yourself saying 'Hold on, didn't we work this way before? What's different about it this time?' Go to your manager and ask questions. You need to know the parameters you will be working in, what the core service/remit/framework/'business plan' is (so many names for the same thing!). But also embrace the change – as they say it is as good as a rest!

Understanding change will enable you to focus on your role, which is assessment of *occupations* and core occupational therapy values; it must always be at the centre of your practice and will keep you grounded when all around is evolving and changing. You will look around and realise that you *are* still working within the social model of disability, legislation relating to our role such as Care Act 2014 *still* applies. The assessment paperwork/recording system/IT/place of work/team may have changed but you will still be focusing on meeting the needs of your service users.

The occupational therapist's role

As an occupational therapist in ASC you will enter a wide range of 'homes', including bungalows, flats, houses, boats or caravans, observing how people interact within them. Some live in extra sheltered housing or supported living units; some temporarily in care homes needing access and/or home visits to facilitate their return home.

You will discuss the relative importance of activities with the individual. Ask 'What is important to you? What will enable you to live well, share and enjoy life?' You will assess their individual needs and functional ability to participate in meaningful activities, while also considering others within the home, the layout, use of areas and so on.

The Care Act 2014 advises the process must be 'person centred', an ethos occupational therapy already advocates. You work with the individual to ensure they are involved in the process and support them to problem solve, have choice and control of solutions to their assessed needs. It is essential you are not focused purely on the individual's disability; they have to be assessed holistically for interventions to work. For example, if the person has difficulties accessing the toilet and bath, there is no point in prescribing a plethora of equipment to facilitate independent bathing if it is going to create barriers for other family members. The equipment will be discarded or rejected and you will be returning to review your original intervention as assessed need was not fully met. What a waste of time and resources – try to keep it simple but effective.

You will also be responsible for *reviewing* manual handling plans, adaptations and equipment, as and when required. This usually includes a reassessment of need 'while you're out there', using the ASC standardised assessment paperwork. This may have a points system connected to a 'care package' allocation or a monetary value associated with a care package. There may also be a risk assessment incorporated into the paperwork.

The occupational therapist role should focus on the 'prevention' and 'personalisation' areas of the Care Act and its incorporation into the ASC assessment. Remember that you are an occupational therapist. Stick the Royal College of Occupational Therapists (RCOT) Code of Ethics on the wall of your office and refer to it whenever in doubt.

There may be pressures for you to work generically and 'sort out' all issues, including ones with no occupational therapy remit. Step back, reflect, be polite and advise there are other resources/professionals/support networks fulfilling this need and refer the individual on to the appropriate service. Signposting is a skill on its own and entails knowledge of services available in your area, eligibility criteria and appropriateness to individual need.

That said, you do work in ASC and are often the first person through an individual's door; you need current knowledge of domiciliary support, respite services, carers' assessments, short-/long-term care, financial assessment and so on – if only to advise these services are available for future consideration. Once equipment and adaptations are in place further services may not be necessary for several years but the person will have the necessary information to refer to in the future.

Breadth of knowledge and signposting skills are particularly useful when you are 'on duty'. Depending upon your team, duty may be solely 'occupational therapy duty' or you may be required to cover duty calls for all team requests. Having a working knowledge of available services, mental capacity assessments and safeguarding on Friday afternoon duty comes in very useful!

The occupational therapy process

Referral

As always this starts with a referral, which may be formal (through a customer service centre) or informal (from a team member). In today's workplace, with the importance of statistics, new referrals and involvements should always be recorded; it is very easy to pop out, 'just to look at some grab rails', unfortunately this won't be recorded or recognised. New referrals will be triaged and then allocated to you by an ASC manager or a senior occupational therapist. Read/discuss the referral thoroughly. Gather information by reading past case notes (if known to the team), research the condition, speak to the referrer if you require further information.

Contact the individual with the need or family member, if appropriate, introduce yourself, explain your role and advise how long the assessment may take. Check their name and contact details (address is especially important). If they live on a long road or in an isolated area ask for a visual reference. In rural areas this may be 'turn right at the large oak tree, turn left at the herd of goats'. If this means nothing to you, be honest; you don't want to be driving/walking/cycling around in the vain hope of finding a herd of goats which may be in for milking.

Ensure they agree to your visit and the assessment. Ask who will be with them during your visit: family carer, large unfriendly dog – all are relevant. Be prepared!

Preparation prior to home visit

Try to make sure you are appropriately dressed for the assessment, review or task you have been asked to do. Check on the internet or a map, where the home is, where it is safe to park (if driving), will there be street lights if the visit is late in the afternoon/early in the morning, is there a key safe? Consider all options. Check for traffic/delays and allow for travel time. While good time-keeping is important, it's better to arrive alive than not at all.

When driving to my visits, I have a pack in the car boot to help meet most situations. Without sounding like a girl guide/scout list it could contain the following:

- mobile phone (with multi-use charger)
- torch (wind-up type/no batteries)
- small slide sheet
- gloves/apron (hygiene)
- toolkit (Allen keys, flat-head and Philips screwdriver)
- 5m and 2m metal tape
- 1m soft tape
- spare trousers
- shoes or wellies depending on season
- sanitising wipes
- stationery
- local map
- waterproof coat
- water.

We know! Bear Grylls would be impressed.

Assessment

Some visits you complete will be joint visits with other professionals but most are completed alone. Ensure you know your lone-working policy and that your team has details of where you are headed, service user contact details and when to expect you back. Some teams operate a 'buddy system' or you may leave details with the duty worker.

TOP TIP

Always be aware of your exits and leave your car facing the direction you intend leaving. There's nothing worse than completing a 25-point turn with several fractious family members watching!

Believe it or not you will already have started your assessment during the earlier information gathering process. Now check the area as you approach. Look for local amenities: shop, clinic, bank, village hall and so on. Think of the individual and their condition as you walk up to the home. Is there a gate, is the path clear, safe, level? What is it made from? Is there room to safely access/egress transport? How wide is the door? How high is the threshold step? Do they have a temporary ramp? Have they come to the door to let you in? How long did it take them? (So much information and you haven't even met them yet.)

Introduce yourself, state your role and purpose for the visit (yes, again), show your ID. Smile. Wipe your feet; you may be asked to remove your shoes (see Jo's tip in Chapter 11, 'Manual Handling'). It's helpful to start with positive small talk: 'What a lovely day/garden/interesting church' – something to break the ice. Their response may also help you ascertain if there is an issue with capacity (more of which later). If you are offered a hot drink, accept and talk to them while they are in the kitchen area, observing movement, cognition and sequencing. You know all this. Observe as they walk and sit/stand.

If others are in the home introduce yourself to them too, ask who they are, do they live there, which roles they complete in the home? and so on. Consider how you would feel if someone sat with their head in paperwork going through a list of questions set by the assessment without any eye contact! Take brief notes as topics are discussed or measurements taken. Keep communication flowing as it allows for exploration yet feels less invasive; use a semi-structured interview technique and open questions for maximum information exchange. Bear in mind the need to change tack, to keep on track or occasionally draw an interview prematurely to a close.

A good starting point is their understanding of the condition/disability causing barriers to function and participation in daily activities. You are completing an assessment *with* a person not *on* a person. Write it in their words, look out for confabulation. Check your paperwork; discuss any specific cultural or religious needs. These may be apparent if you've been asked to remove shoes at the door, for example.

Then move onto their routine. 'What time do you wake? Are you woken by someone? Can you get out of bed on your own?' And so forth. The Person–Environment–Occupation–Participation (PEOP) model seems to work well as a framework in the community, it enables you to remain focused and on task, relating outcomes to a person's wellbeing and ensuring all areas are explored. Observe transfers in all essential areas: bed, toilet, bath, chairs, steps/stairs and access/egress areas of the home. Are they safe? What are the hazards and risks? Is it even possible to complete a functional assessment? Consider end-of-life care.

- A hazard is something which has the potential to cause harm.
- A risk is the likelihood of harm actually occurring.

A matrix with severity on one axis and likelihood of an event occurring on the other on is often used to rate the risk involved for each hazard – low, medium or high.

Adult social care workers try to work with individuals to manage risks but someone living in their own home may choose to continue a risky activity and decline interventions; you may need to complete further risk assessments to see if there is any way to manage identified risks.

Risks include:

- personal injury from falls
- risk to skin integrity
- carer breakdown
- loss of independence
- loss of privacy and dignity
- risk of unintentional self-neglect
- risks linked to medication
- poor nutrition
- risk of social isolation.

You will be reflecting-in-action and have made some decisions on whether the individual is eligible for your service, needs advice and information (such as joint protection or on pacing activities) or is able to self-purchase minor aids/make minor adjustments. Be open and honest about this. You will have to manage expectation and may have to clinically justify, there and then, why you are unable to provide a service.

If you establish eligibility and identify a need, let them know and discuss solutions together. If you need time to consolidate the information, say so, it's OK to say 'I don't know, but I will find out'. Don't forget mandatory paperwork such as consent and capacity forms. Ensure they have your contact details and advise them of any timescales for the assessment paperwork or further visits required. Once the visit has ended, politely take your leave and give yourself a few moments in the car (if you're driving) to evaluate and reflect on the visit.

A word of advice: not all the homes you visit will be cared for, well loved, comfortable, clean and so on. You may not be offered a hot drink on arrival; you may not want to accept a hot drink. All the small talk in your repertoire may not 'break the ice' and there may not be somewhere within the home to sit and amiably discuss needs and solutions.

> Do not try to be super OT and take on all the issues. This is not safe practice and you will only be doing a disservice to the individual and to yourself as a professional.

The individual could possibly be verbally aggressive, rude and judgemental and exhibit challenging behaviours. It could be that your assessment highlights excessive consumption of alcohol or non-prescription medication as the cause of their inability to participate in or access activities of daily living. They may be the victim or perpetrator of domestic abuse. You have a duty to record and report this to your line manager and follow safeguarding policies and procedures – this is where signposting ensures access to the correct service.

Complex core issues

Self-neglect and managing the spectrum of associated needs and adverse health consequences is a core issue for ASC and health services. It involves unpicking why the individual is unable to participate in daily activities, which can be a lengthy, time-consuming process. Self-neglect evolves around five areas: self-care, health, safety, budget and work/leisure. All the areas connect in a negative cycle often resulting in individuals becoming unwell because they have not eaten or taken fluids, then contracting a urine infection, forgetting to take medication, falling because the home is cluttered, or they faint – a real possibility is a fractured hip and hospital admission. If issues relating to self-neglect fail to be addressed and a 'sticking plaster' package of care (three 15-minute calls a day) is put in place, the cycle continues.

It follows that if someone is having difficulty looking after their personal care, they may also have difficulty looking after their home. In extreme cases *hoarding* can result, where someone accumulates excessive amounts of what we may view as 'jumble' but which may have significance to the individual. Or it may be the person simply hasn't the ability to tidy and dispose of items.

Hoarding can be a disorder or a symptom of another condition, such as dementia, depression or obsessive-compulsive disorder. It may be a carer accumulating items whilst attending to the needs of an individual who no longer leaves their bed. It could be someone living alone, no longer able to manage household tasks. Whatever the reason, the hoarding may need to be addressed either before or alongside any possible functional assessment.

From personal experience a home where rooms, hallways and bath are lined with piles of newspaper and magazines makes assessments very difficult. You will probably need to discuss it with co-workers, asking for advice and assistance if necessary.

Hoarding makes cleaning difficult, which can lead to rodent infestations; it can cause 'slips, trips and falls', and it is a potential source of fire. Ensure you know the referral process to your local fire service. They can provide a home fire safety check which is useful in the instances above. Additionally, people on permanent bed-rest who smoke tobacco can be provided with fire retardant bed coverings and emergency plans put in place. The fire service may also be involved in fitting smoke alarms following Telecare provision, checking if someone is sleeping in a room with a gas fire and with evacuation procedures for the plus-sized person.

TIP

As well as networking with the fire service, it is useful to gather information relating to local ambulance services and their response to the plus-sized person. Do they keep a register of residents (who are happy to have their names included on such a register)? Do they have suitable ambulances and equipment to lift or transport larger people in an emergency?

Equally it is also important the individual alerts the services when they move house!

One of the risks mentioned earlier was the risk of social isolation. People who hoard or remain in bed or are unable to mobilise easily outdoors may become lonely and socially isolated. This is where your work in knowing which services are available in your area can come to the fore. Encourage individuals to get out and meet other people or to bring services into their home.

We once found an excellent scheme involving 'exercise to music'. The teacher went into the home and encouraged gentle movement, starting with seated exercises, working towards increased mobility over a six-week period. It was free and the individual was encouraged to join 'exercise to music' classes in their local community, providing an opportunity to increase mobility and function whilst socialising with other people.

Record keeping

If you like spending long periods of time in front of a computer, you will love ASC (or pretty much any occupational therapy role these days)! Whether you offer a service or not, you must record your assessment. Make sure you have training to use the system before starting casework. Use time completing notes and assessments efficiently; this is another opportunity for reflection. As in other settings, records should contain the individual and the occupational therapist's names, dated, and signed if applicable. They should explain concisely what occurred in a way which can be read and easily understood by someone who was not present. They should be factual, reporting what was observed versus what is reported. It may appear rude but in the office I plug headphones in when completing complex assessment paperwork/ notes/planning interventions/completing care planning, to reduce distraction. (The office you will be working in may be open plan and noisy. Do what you need to do to get the task done.)

Equipment

> Please read Chapters 10 and 11 on housing adaptations and manual handling as these will answer questions, in depth and with eloquence, when considering these areas of occupational therapy practice in ASC.

There is so much out there! Equipment is fascinating, ever-evolving, there is a gadget/aid for every conceivable task, well, almost. Attend the Occupational Therapy Show, or its equivalent, but try not to get carried away with sales pitches.

Most local authorities commission a private company to manage equipment stores, giving access to a catalogue of well-tried and tested (contract) items. Visit the store, say hello to the staff; you will be having long conversations with them in the future. Network, network, network. Know your contract items. Try each piece out, take it apart if possible and put it back together. Believe me you will need to be able to do this at some point, usually in the middle of someone's living room floor and invariably with an audience. If you are going to recommend an item, ensure it fits into the environment, their lifestyle, has the correct weight limit and is easy to use for the individual and/or their carer.

> Be aware of medical device alerts and field safety notices, you can sign up to email updates at www.gov.uk/drug-device-alerts.

Consider how it will be fitted and who will fit it. Often you can arrange to trial these in the home prior to provision. Some local authorities have a policy where they do not provide equipment under a set amount as it is reasonable for individuals to use disability allowances/personal independence payments to purchase items. It may sound harsh but a component of this allowance allows for purchase of small aids to promote independent living. You may need to remind the individual of this and signpost them to, for example, disabled living centres, local wellbeing services, Disabled Living Factsheets and so on.The internet provides a wealth of information but as with anything it is a good idea to shop around.

As each individual and their environment is different and if generic contract items have been considered but do not meet need, you will have to research non-contract items where a specialist piece of equipment is provided by a non-commissioned company. They usually have accommodating, knowledgeable advisors/reps who will visit the home with you and complete a *demonstration* of their equipment.

Note we say *demonstration.* They are not there to complete the assessment. That is your job! You have the skills, knowledge, understanding of the individual, how they move, function, their motivation, their environment and how it will all work together. The advisor/sales representative has just walked through the door; they know nothing about the situation, only how the equipment works.

Before supplying equipment a robust justification will be required identifying your clinical reasoning and which should also consider the individual's capacity to accept and appropriately use the equipment. Check the ordering process/requirements with your team manager or senior occupational therapist as this may require authorisation prior to ordering. This usually takes time and may not fit in with urgent needs.

If you consider that the equipment may be restrictive, or you have any doubts about capacity, you must complete a Mental Capacity Assessment. This can lead onto a Best Interest decision being made or Court of Protection involvement to ensure the individual is not deprived of their liberty. Please read Chapter 12 on legislation for further information. It may seem like 'Oh no, not more paperwork/processes'; just remember legislation is there to protect the most vulnerable in our society.

Reviews

The assessment is complete, eligibility has been determined, the care and support plan is in place and services provided – what next? Well, when any service has been provided, an initial review is required. Is it making a positive difference? Safe? Helpful? Is it meeting needs and identified outcomes?

If the answer is yes, then well done you! The casework can be signed off as completed, closed down or placed in the review cycle. The length of time until the next review should be based on your clinical decision. It may be a year; it may be three months or two weeks. It is completed, 'as required'.

If the answer is no, you need to look at an alternative – the toilet seat/frame alone is not providing sufficient support – an integral toilet frame and seat may be needed. Once this is in place and reviewed casework proceeds as above, either full closure or added to the review cycle. Individuals should be kept informed throughout the process and given contact details of your customer service centre (or similar) should they need to get in touch in the future.

Final words

You will undoubtedly have to engage in difficult conversations with individuals. There may be training available. You are required to manage expectations of the service an individual is anticipating and disappointment when an individual does not get what they hoped for. The ASC occupational therapy role is about addressing and meeting *assessed need*, not want. It is a complex role, one in which you will find yourself 'juggling' many tasks. A large proportion of your time will be administrative; there are many processes to safeguard individuals. If you cover a large rural area if possible try to cluster your visits as travelling is time consuming, and remember to allow time in your diary to complete all the other tasks, training, supervision, duty, Christmas parties...

It is essential you network with other occupational therapists working in ASC, as you may be the only occupational therapist in your team and you need to connect with the occupational therapy world for advice, information, reassurance or just to re-engage with professional values. Work collaboratively with the wider multi-disciplinary team: if you look after them they will look after you.

The reward in this role is seeing the progression a person makes because of the advice, support and interventions you provide. This does not only impact on the individual but on families as a whole. By enabling a person to remain in their home, if this is their wish, you promote their wellbeing and feeling of control over key aspects of their life. They become a participant, not a recipient, and you benefit from working in partnership with them.

I hope you have enjoyed this whistle-stop tour of adult social care, and please do take any opportunity to join an ASC team working in the community, providing support and promoting safe and independent living.

10

ADAPTATIONS

Kate Sheehan

A high-quality home adaptation is never an accident; it is always the result of high intervention, sincere effort, intelligent direction and skilful execution; it represents the wise choice of older and disabled people and their families/carers, working alongside building, housing and health and social care professional.

Dr Rachel Russell (2017)

Introduction

Adaptations are a key responsibility of occupational therapists within social care settings. However, there is an increasing requirement for hospital and community-based staff to have some understanding of this complex field of practice. This chapter gives you a whistle-stop tour of knowledge required, enabling you to work in collaboration with clients, surveyors, builders and architects to design and deliver a successful outcome.

Before considering adapting a property it is imperative you look at all other potential options:

- Can you teach a different task technique, which would mitigate the need to adapt?
- Could a piece of equipment enable the task to be completed avoiding the need to adapt?
- Could a minor adaptation support the task being done independently?

Once all the above options have been exhausted then an adaptation can be considered.

The meaning of home

As occupational therapists we need to understand the meaning of a person's home to them and their family, then empower them to make informed decisions about adapting their own home. Recommending major changes facilitating independence can impact on people's emotions linked to their own space and evidence suggests it could significantly impact on whether an adaptation is used. It is therefore critical to discuss *in depth* proposed changes and options available. 'Obliging people to have things they do not like, or about which they have reservations, may result in wholly wasted expenditure' (Heywood 2001, p.45).

Models of practice

As newly qualified occupational therapists you have a deep knowledge of theories of practice underpinning our profession but it can be difficult sometimes to link these into grass roots day-to-day practice.

The model I use on a daily basis, assisting me in my role as a housing occupational therapist, is the Person–Environment–Occupation–Performance model (PEOP), and would strongly advise you spend time reading about this model in depth in Baum and Christiansen (2005).

The model focuses on three areas of knowledge for practice:

- the person (intrinsic factors)
- the person's environment (extrinsic factors)
- the occupations (tasks) a person *needs*, *has* and *wants* to do – the latter as important as the former.

It is client-centred so therapists need to look at everyday occupations as being affected by, and affecting, occupational performance. I will use this approach below to explain how an assessment can be carried out.

There are other theories of practice; as you develop your experience find one which enables you to work in collaboration with clients to achieve the best outcomes.

Assessment

Assessment is key to any successful adaptation and must include the person, the occupation and the environment.

TIP
Every occupational therapist working in housing must invest in a linen or cloth tape and a metal measure, camera and scale ruler.

Person

The first conversation you should have with your client is about their goals, requiring you to listen and understand their reasoning. Although your client may find bathing in a bath difficult, they may wish to continue for a range of reasons:

- They have never showered before.
- They find water on their head disorientating or it provides sensory overload.
- They find a warm bath allows their joints to warm up, improving mobility, making daily activities easier.

You may find a client does not wish to cook and are content with ready meals, the time saved enabling them to spend time with family and friends, or they have never cooked and do not want to learn. Some clients just want to be able to sit at the back door; others may want greater access and use of their garden. Once you have an understanding of their goals, you need to consider how their impairment affects their goals at present.

When designing an adaptation, it is imperative you measure your client and any equipment they use to move around their home (see Figure 10.1).

No one moves in the same way so you must observe how they get around their own home. Remember, they may use different equipment in different parts of the home, for example a wheelchair outdoors, rollator downstairs or commode chair upstairs. You must measure them all; this gives you the knowledge to decide on door and hallway widths, size of lifts, bathrooms or shower areas.

You can use a sketch drawing to do this or your department may have their own standard format.

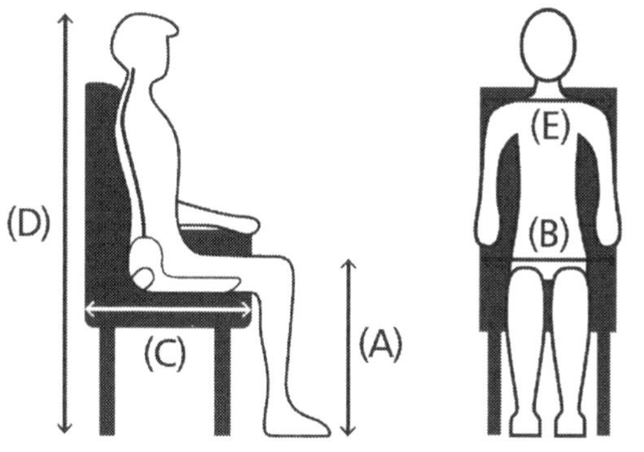

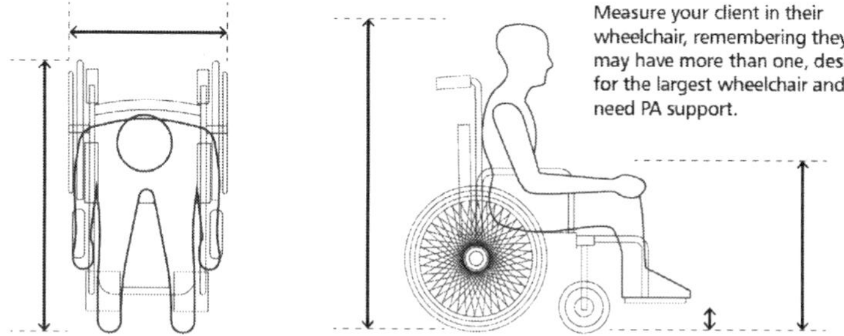

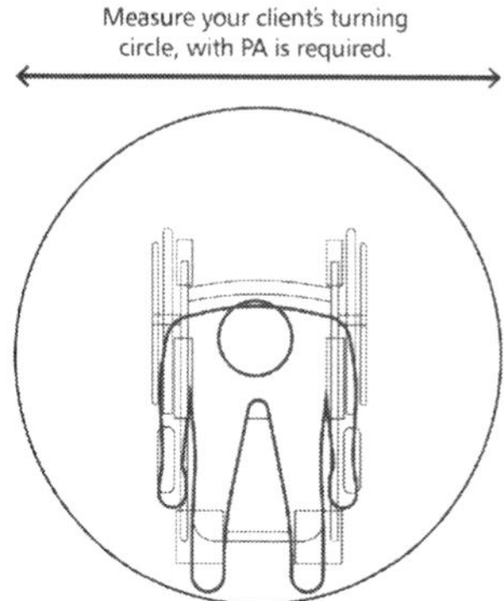

Figure 10.1 Measurements of people and equipment
Source: Kate Sheehan

No two people are the same so you may design something unusable if you do not know what your client can achieve in any range. For example, if you do not know their comfortable reach, you are unable put the shower controls in the right place. Figure 10.2 demonstrates reach in one plane; other examples are available on the internet.

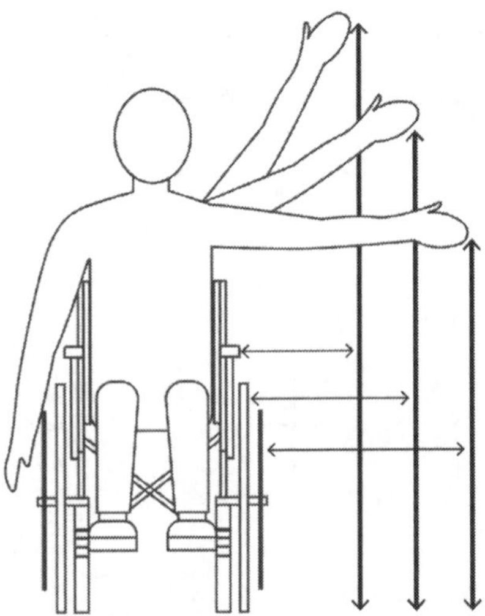

Figure 10.2 Reach when seated

Remember sensory needs; visual and auditory impairments can also be addressed within an adaptation.

Occupation

Having discussed goals with your client, you need to understand how they carry out activities; never presume you know. We all use the toilet in a slightly different way; how they access and use it could be critical to your design. Small details can make the biggest difference; you may be able to get onto the toilet but how do you access and use the toilet paper?

Observation is critical, observe how they do relevant tasks around the home and remember to discuss with carers (paid and unpaid) their level of assistance.

Listen to your client, the primary concern is their view about what they *need* and want to do. Tread carefully. Some people do tasks in a certain way to fulfil cultural or spiritual needs and it is important to be sensitive to these aspects.

Environment/home

The environment does not start at the front door, it starts with the community and area around the property. Bing and Google maps enable you to see the property within context of the community, view the street, the front access and give you a clear idea of plot size. Check the date of maps and videos, these are made at a particular time and things may have changed.

If the property has been sold in the last few years you can sometimes download estate agent plans. It is important to remember they are not always accurate in scale or layout. If this is not possible, you need to do a reasonably accurate sketch drawing (see Figure 10.3). Practise, practise and practise again drawing plans, do your own, friends and family's home layouts. It does not come easy to all, only practising will help.

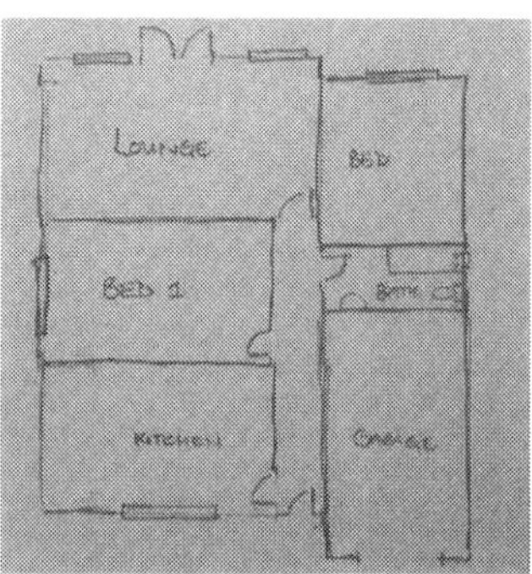

Figure 10.3 Example of a sketched layout
Source: Kate Sheehan

Measure all rooms that impact on your design and mark windows, doors, lights (including switches), sockets and, wherever possible, drainage. Remember, if you are looking at redesigning the bathroom, check where waste and water are as it is costly to move sewage pipes.

There are excellent drawing packages you can use, some paid for and designed specifically for occupational therapists such as *i*dapt

(2017; www.idapt-planning.co.uk). It is easy to use, you can drop PDF drawings into it, make multiple designs for clients and save, share or send to others. There are free drawing packages worth trying if funds are limited.

If you do not have access to drawing packages you must be able to complete scaled drawings of your sketch. Ask experienced colleagues to assist you and to review your drawing as it is essential the design works for your client.

A hand or electronically drawn plan is an excellent tool to help explain the proposed to a client. Figure 10.4 is an example created with *i*dapt. This tool also has a 3D element, which can be a better way of showing a client the final outcome.

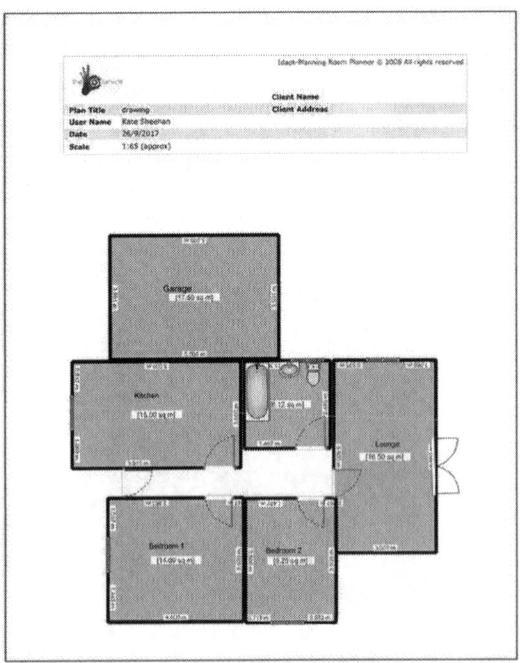

Figure 10.4 Example of a plan created with an electronic drawing package

At the end of any assessment it is important to reflect back information you have received and potential solutions. One of the biggest challenges is managing expectations. Throughout my career I have found two approaches to this situation:

1. *Honesty* – We know that resources are limited, and timescales can be long. Inform clients of issues; effective communication makes for a clearer understanding and better relationship.
2. *Never promise anything* – I often say I need to go away and think, reflect and consult with others before coming up with a solution. This gives time to make an informed decision on potential solutions.

Once you have completed your assessment, write your report with recommendations. These must be linked to clear clinical reasoning, be evidenced from your assessment, linked to legislation and/or evidence available within this area of practice. genHOME is an excellent resource on the RCOT website, available to members, providing recent research on housing adaptations.

Equipment

When designing an adaptation, you need to know which equipment you intend to install, how it will interact within the built environment and how it enables occupational performance. For example, with mobile hoisting you need to allow additional space to manoeuvre the hoist around areas it will be used in and understand methods carers will utilise to move the hoist. For ceiling track or other fixed hoisting systems, think about electrics and where you want the charging point, unless it is a 'track-charging' system.

Consider, when using a tilt-in-space shower commode, do you have space in the shower area for manoeuvring, allowing for carer(s) to assist with personal hygiene?

> **TIP**
> Manufacturers will have technical drawings of the size and details of their products which can easily be downloaded from their website.

Technology is changing very quickly and it is important to keep up to date with new developments. Products which control the environment via units/apps can enable a client to have independent access to managing their environment and thus promote independent living.

Design specification

Once you have agreed your proposed adaptation the next key stage is to write up a clear and concise specification. Most departments will have a proforma or a specific way they construct them, however the key is to remember to put in relevant detail for your client. Use this document to review the finished adaptation and to ensure your brief has been followed.

It should include:

- name and address of the client
- date specification drawn up
- overall aim of scheme – linked to legislation
- drawings if required
- space requirements
- details of requirements for each room, e.g. for bathrooms it should include: type of flooring, lighting, heating and tiles, plus shower area dimensions, type of shower floor (tray or wet floor), position and height of shower controls, riser bar, grab rails and shower seat, also hand basin position, type, height, tap and plug design. For toilets consider style, height, position, type of flush, seat and where the toilet roll holder is located. Include accessories such as shaver socket type and position as well
- a good specification states all electrics should meet the latest Part P Building Regulations
- length and height of grabrails
- length and gradient of ramps.

HINT

If you need to calculate your ramp length, use one of the numerous calculators on manufacturers' websites.

Never send specifications to housing departments or home improvement agencies (HIA) without details. The occupational therapist's role is to clearly specify clients' needs, having completed a comprehensive assessment.

There are excellent design guides to assist in helping plan and design your adaptations, often a local authority will have its own. Remember you are not alone, ask your senior for help, use forums and access the Royal College of Occupational Therapists Specialist Section–Housing for further information.

Communication

To ensure an excellent outcome for an adaptation, a combination of working with the client and the wider design team is required. Get to know your local HIA or surveyors who assist with adaptations. Talk to them, go out on joint visits, ask questions and, most of all, keep each other up to date on progress and agreed outcomes.

Reading and understanding plans

An important skill to acquire is how to read and understand plans. The critical components you need are the ability to:

- read and translate a scaled drawing
- interpret floor and elevation plans
- recognise key architectural symbols and terminology.

I recommend you attend a course introducing you to reading plans. If this is not possible, go out on visits with your local surveyor, asking them to explain their drawings in detail.

TIP

Ask surveyors/architects lots of questions. There is no 'silly' question, just an informed occupational therapist.

Reading and translating a scaled drawing

Various plans are drawn up by architects and surveyors; you need to be able to interpret site and floor plans. Both will have a title block (Figure 10.5), usually situated on the bottom right-hand side of the drawing, and should include the following:

- name and address of the architect or surveyor
- client
- project details

- description of drawing
- drawing number
- drawing date
- drawing author
- scale, including paper size.

C Through floor lift specification added Nov 2017
B Revision to internal access: Bathroom Oct 2017
A Additional window detail added Aug 2017
Rev Description Date
Sheehan
Design Services
Sheehan Design Services Ltd.
Head Office
10 Place Street
Somewhere
County
PQ10 8NJ
DX: **** SOMEWHERE
T: 012280 ******
F: 01280 ******
E: Enquiries@SDS*********
Client
A Person
Project
House Name
House No & Street
Town
County
Postcode
Drawing
Proposed Floor Plans,
And Front Elevation
Ground floor extension to rear
Project No. SDS04913
Design No. 01A
Drawn by KS
Checked By RP
Date 11 Nov 2017
Revision C
Scale @ A1 1:100 1:50
Regional Office
Registered in Country
Registration No:
****
Directors
K Sheehan
B Smith
R Smith

Figure 10.5 Example of title block
Source: Kate Sheehan

Site plans usually show the extent of the site but no surrounding detail and are drawn at either 1:500 or 1:200 scales.

The function of a site plan is to show:

- location of the building
- site topography
- road, footpaths
- planting
- layout of external services, including drainage, water, gas, electrics and telephone
- fencing and walls
- other fixed items, e.g. bollards, lamp posts.

Floor plans show layout of rooms and key dimensions and are drawn at 1:200, 1:100 or 1:50 scales. Their function is to show:

- walls
- windows
- doors
- room designation
- stairs
- fixed furniture
- cupboards/storage
- sanitary fittings.

Elevation plans show the view of a building or room seen from one side, giving a flat representation of a wall or façade. They show:

- doors and their furniture
- height of windows
- position of sanitary items, e.g. height of shower or shower seat
- height of worktops
- height of sockets or switches
- radiators
- pipework.

(Once you have further experience, it is useful to understand block site and assembly plans, especially if you become involved in large extensions or new builds.)

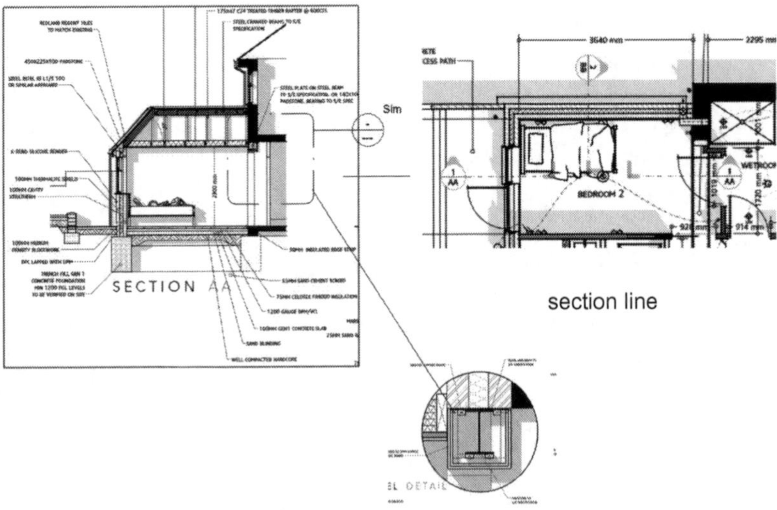

Section & Callout Symbols

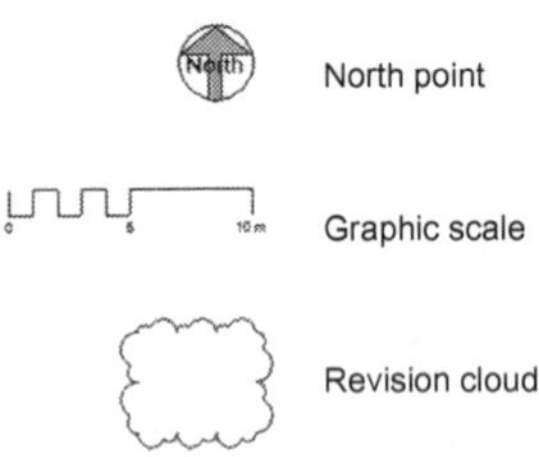

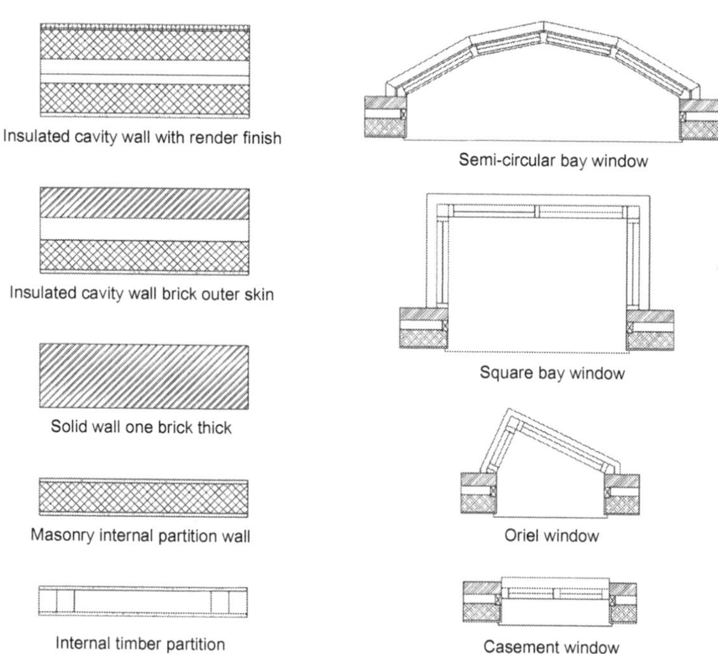

Common wall types

Window types

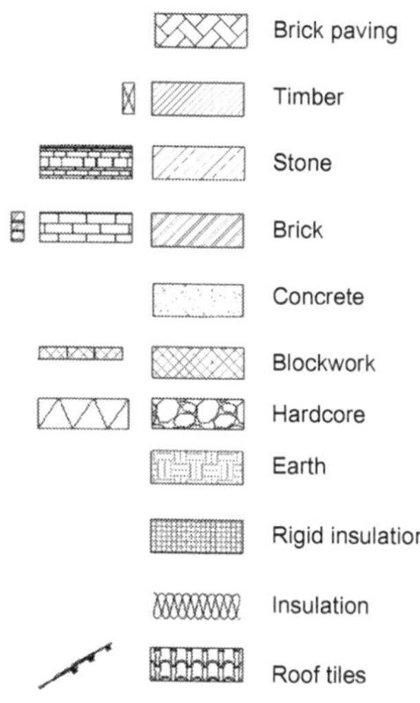

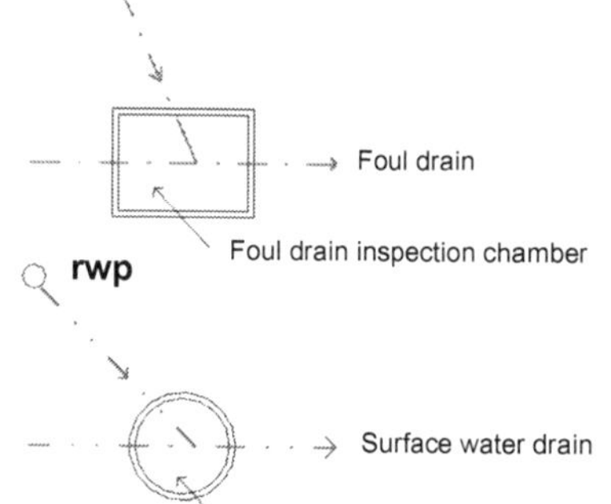

Surface water modular drainage channel

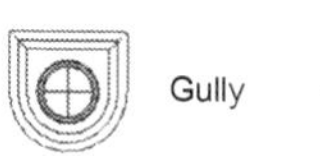

Graphic symbols

Drainage symbols

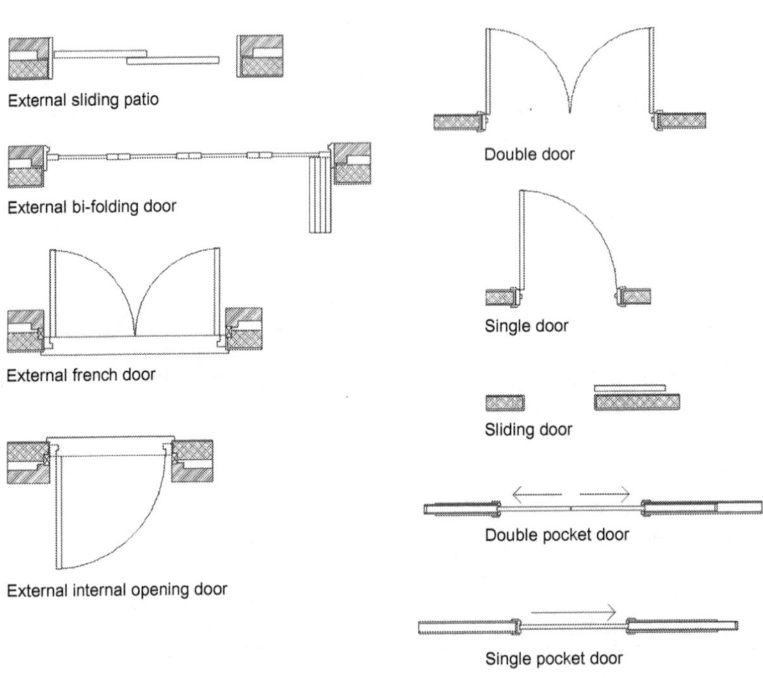
External sliding patio
External bi-folding door
External french door
External internal opening door
Double door
Single door
Sliding door
Double pocket door
Single pocket door
External door types
Internal door types

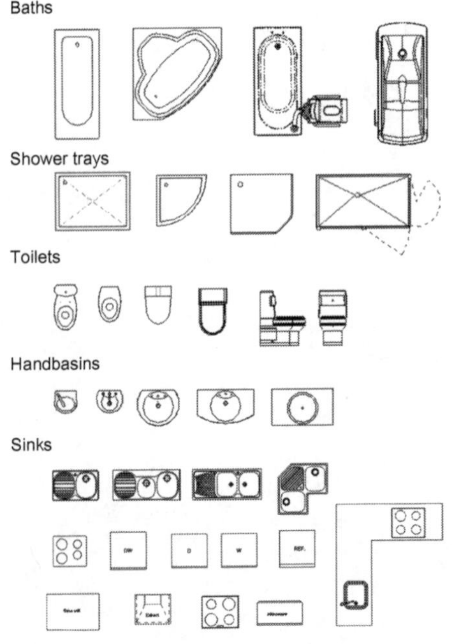
Baths
Shower trays
Toilets
Handbasins
Sinks
DW
D
W
REF.
Bathroom and kitchen appliances

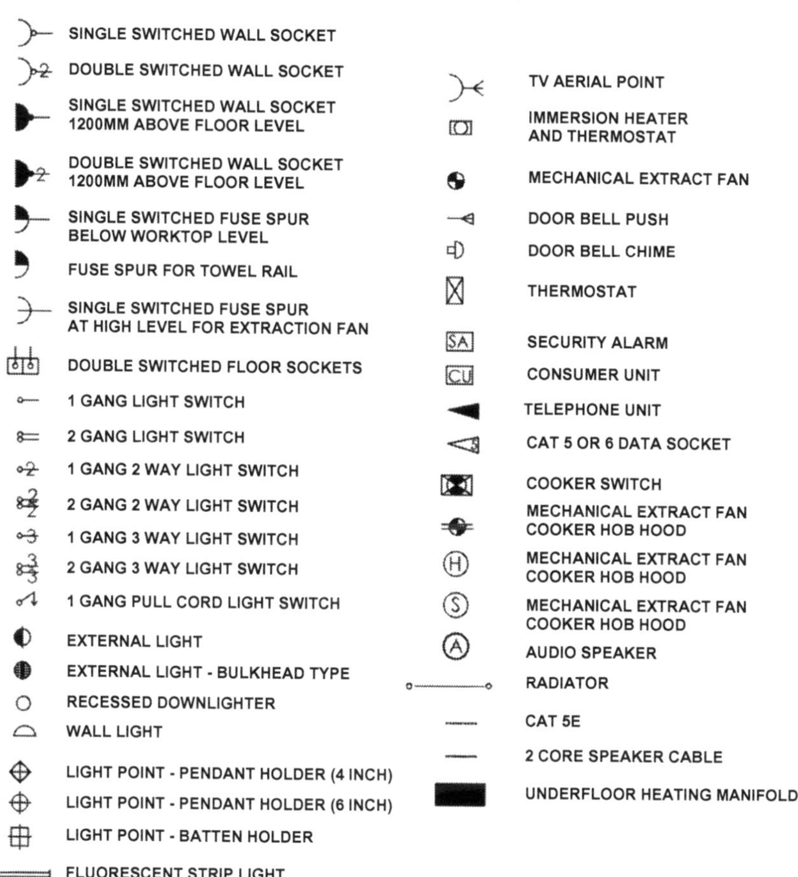

Figure 10.6 Basic key symbols on a drawing
Source: N. Burton, idapt

Remember, when discussing drawings with your client, use layperson's terms not architectural or occupational therapy terms. It is easy to alienate a client with language which is not accessible to them.

Legislation

Legislation is your friend not your foe. It can be used as part of your clinical reasoning and is worth taking time to understand. (Editors' note: Chapter 12 provides detail on other legislation relevant to occupational therapy practice including the Acts listed below. The Housing Grants, Construction and Regeneration Act 1996 and Regulatory Reform (Housing Assistance) Order 2002 are included here in detail due to their direct relevance to this chapter.)

Housing Grants, Construction and Regeneration Act 1996 (Part 1)

This act came into force on 17 December 1996, with further changes introduced in 2008. This Act mandates the Disabled Facilities Grant (DFG), clearly defining the social care occupational therapy role as assessing for need and identifying whether an adaptation is 'necessary and appropriate'. The housing authority has responsibility to decide whether it is 'reasonable and practicable'.

Remember it is not your role to say whether something is 'reasonable', just that it is an assessed need for the modifications recommended.

The DFG is mandatory, that is required by law and compulsory. As long as clients meet the thresholds of 'necessary and appropriate' and 'reasonable and practicable' the local housing authority has to fund works once a client's assessed contribution is paid, this contribution is means tested and at this time this does not apply to those under 18 and on certain benefits. The grant applies to dwellings, qualifying houseboat or park home, the building in which the dwelling or, as the case may be, flat is situated.

> The DFG sits within housing legislation. You cannot use any form of criteria to restrict access.

DFG criteria for a disabled occupant include:

- facilitating access by the disabled occupant to and from the property
- making the property safe for the disabled occupant and other persons residing with them

- facilitating access to a room used, or usable as, the principal family room
- facilitating access to, or providing, a room used or usable for sleeping
- facilitating access to, or providing, a room where there is a lavatory, or facilitating the use of such a lavatory
- facilitating access to, or providing for, a room in which there is a bath or shower (or both), or facilitating their use (the legislation allows for both a shower and a bath if that is the assessed need)
- facilitating access to, or providing, a room in which there is a hand-wash basin, or facilitating its use
- facilitating the preparation and cooking of food. Break down the task of cooking a light meal. It is essential to have access to a sink, fridge, type of oven, storage and preparation area
- improving any heating system in the property or, if there is no existing system or it is system is unsuitable for use by the occupant, provide an appropriate system suitable to meet need
- facilitating the use of a source of power, light or heat, altering its position, access to or control of that source, or by additional means of control
- facilitating access and movement around the property, to enable the occupant to continue in their carer role
- such other purposes as may be specified by order of the Secretary of State
- access to the garden: legislation changed in April 2008, access to gardens became a specific criterion for entitlement where it was 'reasonable and practicable' to do so.

Regulatory Reform (Housing Assistance) Order 2002

Regulatory Reform Orders (RROs) provide councils with more flexibility to tackle private housing in disrepair. The Order repeals much of the existing legislation on discretionary repair and improvement grants, allowing councils to provide assistance for repair, improvement and adaptation through measures such as grants or loans.

The general power under Article 3 of this order enables local authorities (LA) to give discretionary assistance for minor adaptations to either fulfil needs not covered by mandatory DFGs or, by avoiding the procedural complexities of mandatory DFGs, to deliver a much quicker remedy for urgent adaptations. There no restriction on the amount of assistance which can be given.

It also enables the LA to provide assistance to a person to acquire, adapt, repair or demolish dwellings. Top-up assistance to mandatory DFGs can be provided where the local authority takes the view the amount of assistance available under DFG is insufficient to meet the needs of the disabled person and their family.

RROs give local authorities greater powers to provide discretionary assistance, such as:

- low cost loans
- equity release
- funding a move to a more appropriate home.

Each LA will have a published policy on the assistance they will offer.

It is imperative you know this legislation and the key points above. It can form part of your clinical reasoning when writing up your report.

> **TIP**
> To keep up to date on changes and reviews join the RCOT Specialist Section in Housing and also sign up to the Foundations newsletter: www.foundations.uk.com.

Lifting Operations and Lifting Equipment Regulations (LOLER) 1998

With regard to moving and handling equipment it is important to know what duty you have to carers to make sure the environment you are designing meets their needs as well as the clients.

Community Care (Delayed Discharges etc.) Act 2003

Part 2 of this Act provides that any community care equipment and minor adaptations for the purpose of assisting with nursing at home or aiding daily living should be provided free of charge providing the cost is £1000 or less.

Equality Act 2010

The Disability Discrimination Act 2005 has been incorporated into the Equality Act. The definition of disability contained within the Equality Act, crucially, is *linked to a person's ability to carry out ADL* rather than simply to their condition or impairment.

TIP

The Equality Act includes autism as an example of cognitive impairment and therefore a child is eligible under the DFG.

Better Care Fund/Care Act 2013/14

Promotes pooling of resources between health and social care. The Disabled Facilities Grant (DFG) is largely unaffected, although allocation of monies is now through/via the Better Care Fund.

New Approved Part M of the Building Regulations 2015/16

This document lays down minimum requirements required for a new-build dwelling or building in different categories (1, 2 and 3). Category 3 is the one pertaining to wheelchair access.

TIP

Part M contains a useful furniture schedule showing what should be included in each room and furniture sizes. When designing new bedrooms and/or principal family areas it gives an idea of acceptable sizes.

Chronically Sick and Disabled Persons Act (CSDP) 1970

This is currently relevant for children. The provisions are wide ranging and include an assessment for adaptations to the home, or equipment for greater safety, ease or convenience. The Act requires local authorities to inform themselves of the numbers and needs of disabled people in their areas.

Children Act 1989

The act became law in October 1991. This requires local authorities to provide a range of family support services for 'children in need'. This definition includes disabled children.

New-build projects

If you are fortunate enough to have the opportunity to work on the design, specification and build of a new building or dwelling, it is vital you understand the Building Regulations, in particular Approved Document M (HM Government 2016). This gives in-depth detail on what must be achieved, however, it is not a well-defined or easy document to read. The Centre for Accessible Environment and the Royal College of Occupational Therapists Specialist Section in Housing have collaborated to publish the *Wheelchair Housing Design Guide* (2018) which makes clearer the requirements and illustrates additional best practice.

The other key Building Regulations you need to have an awareness of are:

Part B – Fire Safety

Part E – Resistance to passage of sound

Part G – Sanitation, hot water and water efficiency

Part H – Drainage and waste disposal

Part K – Protection from falling, collision and impact

Part P – Electrical safety.

Another core publication to be aware of is BS8300-2:2018, *Design of an accessible and inclusive built environment.* This document, updating the previous version, published by British Standards 'explains how to design, build and manage the built environment in a way that is inclusive. Designing to address and integrate the access requirements of all people, irrespective of their personal circumstances, as part of mainstream design, achieves an inclusive environment which is always preferable to designating separate or specific features' (British Standards Institute 2018).

When involved in the design or critique of a design, make sure you receive a clear and concise brief. This should include:

- details of the target client group
- build construction (on-site or pod)
- budget.

The occupational therapist is key to the usability of the design as they are often the only professional who has insight into how the client group will interact with the built environment.

When reviewing new-build plans, always ask for a full set of plans, including:

- block
- site
- floor
- elevations.

TIP

If you are completing a critique, remember to quote the drawing reference you are commenting on.

Wherever possible try to be part of the on-site team and attend pre-contract and review meetings during the build process. Mistakes made at this point are very difficult to rectify when a building is complete but can be managed during the build if caught early enough. It is critical buildings are constructed to the sizes agreed, as one brick out can make them usable or not.

Just before completion, if a named tenant/owner has been identified for the property, make sure assessed needs such as grab rails are installed to your specification to meet their individual need.

If you wish to become an expert in this area I strongly suggest you attend courses increasing your knowledge on build and construction, regulation and plan critique.

Further information and reading

As your skills develop and you achieve better understanding of the build and construction process, it is worth investing time to improve your knowledge through attending courses. Currently those offered by Viva Access and the Centre for Accessible Environments have excellent content and significant occupational therapy input into their design and delivery.

It is always prudent to keep up to date with equipment and adaptation developments which can be achieved through attending free exhibitions annually.

USEFUL READING

Home Adaptations Consortium (2013) *Delivering Housing Adaptations for Disabled People: A Detailed Guide to Related Legislation, Guidance and Good Practice*. Nottingham: Care & Repair.

Remember clinical practice learning never stops, you will learn daily from your colleagues, your own reading and practice and, most importantly, your client. There is never a one-size-fits-all solution to housing modifications, it is a journey with your client to ultimately meet their own goals.

Remember you are an advocate for your client not a gatekeeper for your employer!

11

MANUAL HANDLING

Jo McKee

Introduction

I recently attended an interview. Part way through, one of the interviewers (the service manager) exclaimed, 'I never realised manual handling was so interesting!' My hope and intention is to share with you, whether you already have experience or are coming to it 'fresh', just how interesting the field of manual handling can be and its relevance to the role of an occupational therapist. There is an expectation as an occupational therapist you will offer expert advice to paid carers and organisations, enable safe handling approaches for informal carers and assess for strategies facilitating independent handling (methods promoting independence). Whilst promoting 24-hour back care, you will need to have an awareness of self, and learn to practice what you preach! There will be times when you work with other skilled professionals in assessing higher risk handling approaches where standard advice is not applicable, such as during rehabilitation or in emergency situations. You will need to have current information and resources at your fingertips to assist and support you with best practice. A resource list (see the 'Professional support' section towards the end of the chapter) will act as a good starting point. I also include 'Top tips', nuggets of information I have shared at training sessions where I have observed a 'lightbulb' moment.

Back care and safer handling

Back pain is classed as a 'musculoskeletal disorder' (MSD). MSDs cover any injury, damage or disorder of joints and other tissues in the back or limbs and have a significant impact on the UK population. Out of the 1.3 million suffering a new or long-standing work-related illness in 2015/2016, 0.5 million related to an MSD (Health and Safety Executive 2016a). The musculoskeletal system is an intricate structure and one of the most vulnerable parts of our body; a subject I anticipate will have been covered in your occupational therapy studies. Adoption of harmful postures such as stooping, bending, kneeling and slouching, aggravated by sustained repetitive or twisting movements, places wear and tear on this intricate structure and can lead to back pain. The risk of injury is further increased if a load is added and/or a sudden, jerky movement completed. The cause of most back pain is unknown and results from cumulative strain, which is a slow build-up of damage to discs, joints, muscles and ligaments. Harmful postures lead to parts of the musculoskeletal system becoming stretched, torn, overworked or, in the case of nerves, trapped. As most episodes of back pain resolve within a short period of time, there is a tendency to ignore signs of damage building up, leading to a condition such as a prolapsed disc.

UNDERSTANDING A PROLAPSED DISC

Place a semi-inflated balloon (or doughnut if feeling particularly messy!) between your hands. Imagine your hands are 2 of the 33 vertebrae in the spinal column. The balloon/doughnut is the disc linking vertebrae together and providing a cushioning effect, a shock absorber between vertebrae. Increase pressure on one side of your balloon/doughnut; this happens to discs during harmful postures such as stooping. (Doughnut users watch out for the jam!) The air in the balloon and the jam represent the nucleus (a gel-like substance) inside the tough outer casing (annulus) of the disc. This casing can burst, the gel leak and touch nerves running from the spinal cord, triggering pain.

In your career you will meet carers who advise that they hurt their back when gardening or bending. As professionals involved in back care an important message we need to get across is that the *onset of pain* may have been at the point of bending or gardening, the *injury* is due to a lifetime of harmful posture. It is also worthwhile stressing to carers the effects of back pain and how disabling it can be. Unpaid carers are an 'at risk' group with both physiological and psychological factors involved. BackCare, a national charity educating the public in ways of preventing and alleviating back pain, cite on their website that 1 in 10 of the UK population are unpaid carers, and 70 per cent already suffer with back pain. Unpaid carers may have a loving and altruistic approach and do not value themselves in the equation. However, who will look after the individual if the carer is unable to do this themselves?

TOP TIP

When assisting a person to move, imagine you have a beam of light shining from your belly button. If your hands are not in the beam, the likelihood is you are twisting.

We also need to look after ourselves as health professionals. We too have the same intricate spinal structure. Back care should not be kept for the workplace but considered in all of our activities of daily living. Consider a shopping trip. How do you pack the boot, without thinking at all or do you put the lighter items to the back and heavier to the front? Do you overreach when lowering bags into the car boot or do you adjust? Do you use large 'bags for life' or divide the load and use smaller bags? I have got over the fact I may get odd looks going down the food aisle; I relax my knees and lead with an upward movement of the head when initiating motion of my trolley!

It is not only when we are active we need to consider back care but also in the sedentary lifestyles we lead. I would say regrettably I spend more time sitting in front of a computer as an occupational therapist than I do being active. Consider your workstation. Are you maintaining a good posture? If not, do you need a Display Screen Equipment (DSE) Work Station Assessment? Do you drive when you are at work?

BackCare offer good guidance and fact sheets on their website (see 'Useful websites' at the end of the chapter) in relation to the above.

Short (micro) breaks at regular intervals, when you move about, allow your body to change position and to recover. When moving, our muscles contract, tighten and relax. This action helps to pump blood and other fluids containing oxygen and nutrients around the body to muscles and waste products away from them. During harmful postures certain muscle groups work harder and tense up, restricting blood flow.

For example, when stooping over a bed, muscles in the back of our legs and lower back become tense. They have to work hard, stopping our body from toppling over as we move far out from our central line of gravity. There are other recognised lifestyle choices helping to maintain a healthy back. These include exercising regularly but safely; eating a healthy diet; carrying your bag (such as a rucksack) on both shoulders rather than on one; choosing not to smoke (this can reduce blood supply to the intervertebral discs); maintaining a healthy weight; selecting a bed offering the correct comfort and support and, finally, finding ways to manage stress.

TOP TIP

Flex your fingers into a fist and hold for about 60 seconds (less if it becomes uncomfortable). During this time observe changes occurring in the skin and sensations you feel. Skin may change colour. It may feel hot or cold. Tingly? These changes are effects of restricted blood flow to this area of the body. Now release the fist hold. What do you observe? How long does it take to return to your normal state? This is the recovery period. Often our muscles do not get the required time to fully recover.

So let's clarify what manual handling is. Over the years different terminology has appeared from 'moving and handling' to 'safer handling' to 'assisting a person or object to move'. These are defined in the Manual Handling Operations Regulations (MHOR) 1992 as 'any transporting or supporting of a load (including the lifting, putting down, pushing, pulling, carrying or moving thereof) by hand or bodily force'. The load can be an object, person or animal. A load is defined in the *Oxford Dictionary of English* (Stevenson 2010) as 'a heavy or bulky thing that is being carried or is about to be carried'.

How do we define heavy or bulky? *Manual Handling Operations Regulations 1992 Guidance on Regulations* from the Health and Safety Executive (HSE) (2016b) is a useful publication offering guidance on risk filters, and when weight of a load is an important factor to consider. The shape, size and nature of a load will also affect whether it is carried away from the body, placing a greater strain than holding it close. It may be harder to get a secure hold of the load, vision may be restricted due to its size and shape or it may be unwieldy and/or unpredictable.

When preparing to move an object or person it is important to adopt good handling techniques if there are no alternative risk-reduction measures, such as the use of lifting equipment or modifications to task, load or environment. Consider, prior to moving, whether it is possible to move a load in an alternative way, such as by sliding or rolling. You may wish to rock an inanimate object from side to side to get an idea of its weight. Are there ways to reduce the size and shape of the load before lifting? Keep any lifting to a minimal distance and range. There may be times when you need to lower the load, adjusting part way through a lift, to reposition self and load. Ensure you remain working within a stable base and have a secure hold.

There is no single way to assist a person to move, and there are different movement methods to consider, each with their own merit. The HSE commissioned the Institute of Occupational Medicine to produce a research report entitled *The Principles of Good Manual Handling: Achieving a Consensus* (Health and Safety Executive 2003). This presented the outcomes of a 'Delphi exercise' undertaken to establish scientifically-based principles for manual handling training. A series of 11 principles was identified relating to two-handed symmetrical lifting. These are:

- Think before you lift.
- Keep the load close to your waist.
- Adopt a stable position.
- Ensure a good hold on the load.
- At the start of the lift, moderate flexion (slight bending) of the back, hips and knees is preferable to fully flexing the back (stooping) or the hips and knees (squatting).
- Don't flex your spine any further as you lift.
- Avoid twisting the trunk or leaning sideways, especially while the back is bent.
- Keep your head up when handling.
- Move smoothly.
- Don't lift more than you can easily manage.
- Put down then adjust.

The report recognised there are anomalies, two-handed symmetrical lifting is not always possible, and offers guidance applicable in non-standard lifting situations.

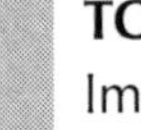

TOP TIP

Imagine you are sitting a perching stool to understand what is meant by 'soft knees', 'relax down' or 'moderate flexion'.

It is important to recognise these principles as underpinning movement methods which you will use in your handling plans. These should also apply in everyday life for continued back care. You may work with carers who have attended manual handling training and are aware of the principles or with families who have received no formal training. It is often unpaid carers who undertake manual handling facilitating personal care on their own. These same carers will be pushing the person they care for in a wheelchair throughout the day. It strikes me it is often these people who are more susceptible to injury resulting from assisting a person to move. Although equipment can be offered to reduce the level of handling taking place, they also need to be made aware of the principles for safer handling to use equipment efficiently and safely.

Legislation and risk assessment

As a healthcare professional, legislation applies to your role. It may appear as a very 'dry' topic, so a good approach to take is to treat it as your friend. Legislation considered in this chapter is specific to manual handling. Further information can be found in Chapter 12 'Legislation'.

Manual handling legislation can be split in to three main categories. European legislation is intended to harmonise standards throughout the European Union (EU). It is achieved through a directive each European member state is required to assimilate into their own legislation. European directives brought about important changes to UK health and safety statute law in 1992. As we embark on the Brexit journey, the next few years will be an interesting time. It is unknown what regulatory changes may occur, if any!

Statute law, also referred to as written or criminal law, has been the main source of UK legislation in modern times and is designed to ensure fairness. A breach of statute law is an offence, leading to prosecution through the criminal courts. Common law, or civil law, provides individuals via the legal system compensation/redress, cases argued on their own merits and expert evidence sought to prove which standards are reasonable.

The Health and Safety at Work Act 1974 (HASAWA) is often referred to as umbrella legislation in terms of other UK manual handling legislation. It is the basis of UK health and safety legislation and details employer and employee rights and requirements regarding safety in the workplace. It places a duty on all employers 'to ensure, so far as is reasonably practicable, the health, safety and welfare at work' of all their employees.

Duties of employers include ensuring safe systems of work are in place to establish a safe place of work and environment. To support this, there must be a hard copy safety policy and employees must be supported by training, information and appropriate levels of supervision. Additionally, associated items and substances must be stored, maintained and transported and handled in a safe manner.

It is important to remember the Act also places duties on employees, who must take responsibility for their own health and safety (within reason) but also have responsibility for the outcome of their actions (or omissions) on others. There is also a duty to cooperate with their employer on health and safety matters and they should not interfere with or misuse health and safety provisions.

The Management of Health and Safety at Work Regulations 1999 (MHSWR) were introduced to support the Health and Safety at Work Act 1974 and clearly explain how safe systems should be implemented and managed in the workplace. The main requirement on employers being to appoint competent persons to complete assessments of risk for employees and others affected by their work activity. Those with five or more employees are required to record the significant findings of the risk assessment.

Other provisions under the Regulations include health monitoring for employees, procedures to manage serious incidents and where there is imminent danger, and to support new employees through induction, assessing their capabilities and providing instruction. There are also duties in regard to age-related needs (young/old) and for pregnant women and new mothers.

Under the Regulations, employees must inform the employer of identified hazards and follow any instructions given.

A definition of 'cooperate' in the *Oxford Dictionary of English* is 'work jointly towards the same end' (Stevenson 2010). The word 'cooperate' appears frequently in the above legislation. It is quite clearly a two-way process. When applying to practice, employers have a duty to provide systems to keep you safe in the work environment. Our work environment is extremely varied. You may work on a rehabilitation ward, residential unit, school or service user's home, in the company of an occupational therapy colleague or other healthcare professional, carer (paid or unpaid) and the person you are assisting to move. Legislation requires you to take reasonable care of your own and their safety, not only through what you do but also what you do not do. Your employer has a requirement to provide you with the 'tools' you need to carry out your job safely, such as a health and safety policy and procedures, and provision of necessary training. However, as previously mentioned, it is a two-way process, you have a responsibility to report if you are not provided with these tools or if they are inadequate.

MHOR 1992 came into force on 1 January 1993 implementing European Directive 90/269/EEC4 on the manual handling of loads into UK law, supplementing other occupational health and safety legislation. The Regulations require employers to:

- *avoid* the need for hazardous manual handling 'so far as is reasonably practicable'
- *assess* the risk of injury from any hazardous manual handling that cannot be avoided
- *reduce* the risk of injury from hazardous manual handling 'so far as is reasonably practicable'
- *review* the assessment if new information comes to light or if there has been a significant change in the manual handling operations.

An employer's duty to avoid manual handling or reduce the risk of injury is determined by what is considered 'reasonably practicable'. It does not mean a blanket ban on lifting, as this would be unlawful, it means balancing level of risk against measures needed to control risk.

Identification of risk should not be influenced by available resources; risk-reduction actions can be *balanced* against resources, considering money, time, trouble and whether the need to take action would be grossly disproportionate to level of risk. For example, you may find the most expensive option is not reasonably practicable but the cheaper option is a viable and safe alternative.

Each manual handling task needs to be individually assessed, a reasonably practicable solution in one circumstance may not be considered the same elsewhere.

What is meant by risk assessment? It is a term you will hear quite often in your occupational therapy career and not always in reference to manual handling. Risk assessment is a method for weighing up risk. 'Risk' is the likelihood of harm or injury occurring. We complete risk assessments informally, such as when crossing roads, preparing to cross, we check if the road is busy. Do we have a clear view of oncoming cars? Are there pot-holes in the road? All of these are considered hazards. Hazards are anything causing/that could cause injury or harm. Employees are required to assist in identifying, removing or avoiding hazards if possible, reporting them to their line manager as soon as possible to enable a risk assessment to be undertaken.

Where risks are associated with manual handling, a risk assessment must be carried out in a particular way as outlined by MHOR 1992. You will probably come across the acronym *TILEO* when completing a manual handling risk assessment as we consider the *T*ask, *I*ndividual capability, *L*oad, *E*nvironment and *O*ther factors. An ergonomic approach ensures the task is fitted to the person and not the other way around.

DID YOU KNOW?

ATMs were originally designed in the UK to give you cash before returning your bank card. This was reviewed after incidents where users forgot to collect their card. Their goal was to withdraw money, the end goal being to receive cash. Users considered the task completed when in receipt of cash, leaving without the card. An ergonomic approach was utilised, bringing the task flow in line with users' goals; cards are now received before cash.

Task

We need to consider which safer handling principles are not being complied with, asking which harmful postures and movements are used? Do they involve holding or manipulating loads away from the trunk or excessive lifting, lowering, carrying, pushing or pulling? Is there exposure to jerky, sudden or unpredictable movement? Are there sufficient recovery periods between movements? You may find you are able to reduce the risk of injury by changing the task layout.

Individual capability

In terms of a manual handling risk assessment we consider the capability of those being assisted to move. Do they have a long-standing medical condition/injury restricting them? Do they have a disability affecting movement? Are they pregnant? Does their weight/health restrict their own functional abilities? Are they a person predisposed to musculoskeletal injury? Does the task require working at unusual height or increased strength?

Load

The terminology is unfortunate, here the 'load' refers to the person being assisted to move. Your assessments need to consider their weight, abilities, unpredictable movements and behaviours. How do they communicate, and how can they be communicated with?

Environment

Where is the task taking place? Is there adequate space to ensure poor posture is not adopted? Are floors level, uneven or slippery? Is lighting and room temperature sufficient?

Other

Consider anything else affecting the activity. Is movement or posture hindered by personal protective equipment or by clothing? Have near misses/accidents been reported? Is a staff rota in place to facilitate recovery periods?

It is important to have sufficient detail clearly showing links between hazard identification and risk-reduction measures. Clinical reasoning must be evidenced as a part of your assessment process. As an occupational therapist, you need to evidence reasoning for risk-reduction measures you are recommending. Remember occupational therapy core business includes enabling independence, provision of equipment and adapting the environment.

For example, you may observe a manual handling activity carried out on a box-base divan bed placed against the wall. Your hazard identification highlights the carer is having to stoop and overreach several times a day, ten minutes at a time, to assist with personal care. They dual-task by supporting the person in a side-lying position, carrying out personal care, adopting twisting movements. Your risk-reduction measures may include equipment enabling the person to independently move on the bed. By recommending equipment such as a height-adjustable profiling bed and positioning wedge, carers can adjust the bed to a suitable working height while the person is supported in side-lying. Another risk-reduction measure may be to modify the environment: positioning the bed away from the wall facilitates access from either side. Completion of a handling plan accessible to all carers will be another risk-reduction measure.

Despite a review date on manual handling risk assessments, it is still important to complete an 'on the spot' risk assessment prior to an activity as there may be changes occurring on that day at that time. This includes a pre-use check of equipment and environment, evaluating the wellbeing of people involved, including the person you are assisting to move. Inform your line manager if there are changes affecting the way the person is to be moved, this ensures a review is completed. Be familiar with the procedure to be followed in emergency situations.

In terms of manual handling of people there are two types of risk assessment needed: generic, for the setting, and individual. Last year I completed a generic risk assessment for our local swimming pool. For this I considered the user population, training needs of staff, the environment, identifying hazards and if equipment in place met need. I reviewed operating procedures and moving and handling required in an emergency. A completed risk assessment was forwarded to the swimming pool committee with recommended actions and review date.

Individualised risk assessment is specific to a person and should consider manual handling needs as part of their care plan. It is probably the manual handling assessment you will be asked to complete as an occupational therapist, and you will need to review it as their condition changes. The handling plan formed from the findings of your risk assessment will identify when manual handling is needed, recommended movement methods, the number of competent persons required and person specific information. It provides equipment details and how they are used, such as loop configuration on slings. Individual information such as whether the person has a preferred side to be rolled on to or approached from must be included.

During the pool assessment risks were identified associated with use of the pool slide and inflatables. These could be avoided by banning their use. *Why didn't I take a risk-adverse approach and recommend a blanket ban on slides and inflatables?* The answer is that when completing a risk assessment we need to take all factors into consideration. In this situation it included the wishes and expectations of those using the pool facility. It is a fun pool, having had these facilities for many years, resulting in community expectation. A balanced approach was taken, safe systems put in place, managing identified risks with use of slides and inflatables.

Service users and families have expectations of what is acceptable. When completing a manual handling risk assessment there is a need to consider welfare and human rights legislation, including the Human Rights Act 1998, Mental Capacity Act 2005 and Equality Act 2010; more information can be found in Chapter 12, 'Legislation'.

Manual handling assessments can be complex. You may work with individuals where, considering risk reduction to a reasonably practicable level, you identify an appropriate movement method. However, the individual and or carers disagree. In these circumstances a balanced decision-making approach is required. Collaborative working with other involved professionals ensures all avenues are explored. There may be circumstances where paid carers might work at higher but not unacceptable levels of risk to meet identified needs. The importance of a robust risk assessment in such complex cases cannot be stressed enough!

Other professionals can be responsible for completing a manual handling risk assessment. I have worked with colleagues including nurses, physiotherapists and ergonomists particularly skilled in this area.

As occupational therapists, our skills and knowledge lend themselves well to this task. We are familiar with activity analysis required to break down the task. We are good problem solvers, provision of equipment and adapting environments are integral parts of our practice. There are not always obvious solutions to complex risk assessments but I would argue our skill base is a perfect match!

Assisting a person to move

Reading this article was a turning point in my own practice: 'Manual handling questions' (MHQs) by physiotherapist April Brookes (2008) concisely frames the assessment and decision-making process we utilise before assisting a person to move. MHQs adopts a logical principle-based approach seeking to maximise the service user's functional ability and independence. There is a hierarchy of five questions to consider:

1. What is the normal movement for this task?
2. Can I teach the person to do this unaided?
3. If not completely unaided, is there equipment available which would mean the person could do this for themselves?
4. If unable to perform the task themselves, what is the minimum of assistance one and then two people can give (a) without equipment and (b) with equipment?
5. Are there unsafe ways of doing this I must avoid? (If so, what are they?) (Brookes 2008)

The first question considers normal movement patterns. If you are not familiar with these, complete the task; for example, rolling in bed, then think about how you achieve this. Alternatively, observe someone carrying out the task. Familiarity with normal movement patterns may be key when re-educating those you are assisting to move to promote independence.

If the person is unable to complete the task unaided, it is time to consider whether equipment can assist. Equipment assisting sit-to-stand transfers ranges from consideration of the chair used. If the person can stand, weight-bear or move laterally, then a transfer board could be considered. If the person is able to weight-bear but not take steps you may consider equipment to facilitate a pivot transfer such as a Patient Turner or more flexible options such as an Arjo Stedy or Re-Turn. If they are unable to move from sit to stand but can weight-bear, you may consider a standing hoist, also referred to as an active lifter. If unable to weight-bear, a passive lifter such as a mobile or ceiling track hoist is recommended. There are numerous aspects to consider when assessing for a hoist and sling. The HSE offers guidance in their article *Getting to Grips with Hoisting People* (2011), including a flowchart assisting decision-making in this process.

It may be identified that more than one handler is required to reduce the risk of injury when assisting the person to move. However, a second handler can introduce additional factors you need to consider. When the need for two handlers has been identified it is important to specify their responsibilities in the handling plan and for them to be familiar with this prior to assisting the person to move. You may find in practice that when reviewing a manual handling plan you identify there is no longer a need for two handlers or that handling can be achieved by one handler and alternative equipment.

My benchmark during assessment is 'How would I like to be moved?' 'How would I like my child to be moved?' 'How would I like my mother to be moved?' I think I would prefer a one-to-one approach, dignity shown, engagement between carer and person being moved, with movements carried out as safely as possible. We come back to balanced decision-making and compromise.

With regards to provision of equipment, manufacturer's guidance in the form of manuals offers accompanying product-specific instruction and information. Some manuals can be extremely informative. You will work with product assessors (reps), who have detailed knowledge of their products. Having worked in this role for several years, completing on average five sling assessments a day, I had opportunities to have 'lots of goes', thus gaining experience. As an occupational therapy practitioner we do not generally have these opportunities. Remember, although we can benefit from the knowledge of product assessors, at the end of the day it is the occupational therapist's responsibility to provide *clinical reasoning* regarding equipment provision.

A word of caution. If using equipment or a movement method you are not familiar with, it is reasonable to look online for guidance. Over the years I have seen some excellent online tutorials and some causing concern, offering in my opinion poor practice. I suggest using these as a learning opportunity, critically appraise movement methods and do not just accept what you see.

Equipment issued to assist with manual handling tasks needs to be identified if it falls under the Provisions and Use of Work Equipment Regulations (PUWER; 1998) or Lifting Operations and Lifting of Equipment Regulations (LOLER; 1998).

How the Lifting Operations and Lifting Equipment Regulations Apply to Health and Social Care (HSE 2012) offers clarity on the requirements of LOLER in these settings and with which types of equipment. Equipment categorised as lifting equipment is subject to a six-monthly LOLER inspection completed by a person competent in relation to the equipment. Equipment not falling under LOLER but used for work purposes, for example for a paid carer assisting a person to move, is subject to a schedule of regular maintenance under PUWER.

When answering question 5 of the MHQs we need to understand what high-risk handling is. Certain handling activities were referred to as 'banned'. This takes us back to the idea of blanket terminology. No legislation has been introduced stating certain movement methods are banned. However, when we consider the 'task' part of certain movement methods we can identify that they result in high-risk handling. Best practice literature such as *The Guide to the Handling of People* (Smith 2005) has a chapter with an evidence-based review on handling activities previously viewed as controversial, offering support evidencing their high-risk status.

Wherever you work there is policy and procedure in relation to manual handling. Familiarise yourself with it as part of your induction into the workplace. One topic usually included is information on appropriate dress. It is widely considered that 'suitable footwear' constitutes supportive, covered flat footwear. Policy for your workplace may be more specific. I have experienced situations when undertaking a manual handling assessment when I have been asked to remove my shoes. To save awkward moments I now keep appropriate shoes in my car, these for indoor only. Guidance may include no jewellery or a requirement for short fingernails. This is not only there to protect you but also the person you are assisting to move. It would not be pleasant to have jewellery digging in to your back or gel nails caught whilst a sling is fitted.

Professional support

An important point to remember, whatever stage you are at in your career, is the support of others. Occupational therapists can often be viewed as the 'expert' in manual handling, which can be a daunting position when newly qualified. Even when you have experience under your belt there will be occasions when there is unrealistic expectation that you will have an immediate solution pleasing all involved. To reiterate a point already made, manual handling can be complex and collaborative working is key.

You may find yourself part of a large occupational therapy team, working independently, or part of a multi-disciplinary team as the only occupational therapist. If peer support with specialist knowledge is not readily available, there are other avenues to explore. There will be groups meeting in your area focusing on manual handling and leading to great networking. The National Back Exchange (NBE) has regional groups around the country; their mission statement is 'to develop, disseminate and promote evidence based best practice in moving and handling'. They also publish a quarterly journal, *The Column*, and hold an annual conference. Members have a wealth of experience, knowledge and a willingness to share. It may be that you prefer a more localised approach and wish to attend a special interest group in your area or consider mentor support through a one-to-one approach. You can also identify best practice in literatures such as the Handling of People (HOP) book (Smith 2013) and manual handling guidance available on the Royal College of Occupational Therapists (RCOT) website. The NBE have produced 'Professional Series' books specific to areas of work including paediatrics and bariatrics. The HSE is the UK government body responsible for enforcing health and safety at work legislation, also offering advice on health and safety issues and guidance on legislation through their website.

Conclusion

Writing this chapter has felt like a whistle-stop tour on a complex subject. There are no set answers or solutions. I hope the information shared empowers you to make informed choices, be able to demonstrate evidence-based decision-making and facilitate the problem solving approach required in this complex field. It is an interesting area of work as two situations are never the same. As you develop and gain experience, you will be applying knowledge to new situations but there will always be something making each scenario unique and specific to the person you are working, requiring a person-centred approach.

USEFUL WEBSITES

Back Care: www.backcare.org.uk
Health and Safety Executive: www.hse.gov.uk
National Back Exchange: www.nationalbackexchange.org.uk
Royal College of Occupational Therapists: www.rcot.co.uk

12

LEGISLATION

Julia Badger and Kate Sheehan

Additional information provided by Viva Access (www.viva-access.com), a specialist training and access consultancy offering a range of courses on adaptations.

Legislation can be considered as being a bit like Marmite, people either love it or hate it. (Julia used to be in the 'hate' camp, mainly finding the language and legal jargon confusing – but not any longer.) Taking time to research, study and attempt to understand often convoluted language will hopefully encourage 'haters' to embrace legislation and use it when justifying or explaining actions or interventions as part of clinical reasoning. Obviously, please read up on any legislation connecting to the occupational therapy role or path you intend to take, but to save you time we have broken down some of the core legislation mentioned in the chapters in this book.

Legislation refers to the process of enacting statutory laws or to the set of statutory laws in a state; passed by a legislature and, in some cases, also confirmed by the executive. When a bill becomes a law, the law is said to be 'promulgated' or 'enacted'. We need legislation in place to ensure society runs smoothly, equitably, fairly and safely, protecting you as a professional and the people you work with. Without legislation there would be chaos and disorder. You will see from Table 12.1 how just a small sample of legislation runs through all areas of practice.

(Not all acts are expanded on in this chapter and information provided is just an overview. The Care Act and Mental Capacity Act have more detail due to their prominence. Research and reading are essential to ensure you understand the implications and intricacies in application to practice.)

Table 12.1 Summary of legislation cross-referenced with relevant areas of OT practice

Legislation	Year	Relevant chapters							
		4 NHS	5 Paeds	6 MH	7 LD	8 CWD	9 ASC	10 Adaps	11 M&H
Care Act	2014	✓	✓	✓	✓	✓	✓	✓	✓
Mental Capacity Act	2005	✓	✓	✓	✓	✓	✓	✓	✓
Housing Grants, Construction and Regeneration Act	1996					✓	✓	✓	
Lifting Operations and Lifting Equipment Regulations	1998	✓	✓		✓	✓	✓	✓	✓
Community Care (Delayed Discharges etc.) Act	2003	✓	✓	✓	✓	✓	✓	✓	✓
Equality Act	2010	✓	✓	✓	✓	✓	✓	✓	✓
Better Care Fund	2013 /14	✓	✓	✓	✓	✓	✓	✓	
Chronically Sick and Disabled Persons Act	1970	✓	✓	✓	✓	✓	✓	✓	✓
UN Convention on the Rights of the Child	1989		✓			✓		✓	
Children Act	1989	✓	✓	✓	✓	✓		✓	
Human Rights Act	1998	✓	✓	✓	✓	✓	✓	✓	✓
Provisions and Use of Work Equipment Regulations	1998	✓	✓	✓	✓	✓	✓	✓	✓
Autism Act	2009	✓	✓	✓	✓	✓	✓	✓	
Freedom of Information Act	2000	✓	✓	✓	✓	✓	✓	✓	✓
Data Protection Act	1998 2018	✓	✓	✓	✓	✓	✓	✓	✓

Care Act 2014

Though lengthy and containing many chapters and sub-chapters, the Care Act 2014 is a single law making clear what care should look like and how it should be delivered for those who need care, carers and people working in health and social care settings. Prior to this a plethora of legislation was in place, complicated and confusing enough for managers of care services and systems, let alone individuals seeking care and support.

It has made major changes to the way local authorities provide social care and promotes coordination with relevant partners such as clinical commissioning groups (CCGs). The Care Act is mainly about people 18 years and over who need care and support. It also includes young people age 16+ as part of the 'Transitions' component. The act focuses on person-centred care and wellbeing, with clear areas covering prevention, accessing adaptations and equipment which are particularly useful for occupational therapists:

- *Wellbeing* – the wellbeing principle puts wellbeing at the heart of interventions or interactions. It guides the local authority to promote wellbeing in all areas of care and support. (Think about person-centred practice and inclusion.)
- *Prevention* – this theme covers a wide range of care and support services and focuses on early intervention to enable people to maintain or regain confidence and skills. It promotes health, wellbeing and independence. (Use this area of the Act as support for equipment, aides and adaptations especially with regards to futureproofing.) Prevention should be seen as an ongoing process and not as a single intervention.
- *Assessment and eligibility* – the local authority has a duty to provide a holistic needs assessment, to be completed with the person in a collaborative way, taking into consideration how support networks and the community can contribute to achieve outcomes. The assessment should include leisure/work as well as the standard list of activities of daily living. An eligibility threshold determines whether a person has eligible needs; the Act states the person must be informed if they are eligible for care and support or not.

- *Integration* – health, care and support services must work together to provide high quality care. The aim of integration is to prevent services working in silos and reduce the frustration arising from disjointed services as poor care impacts negatively on health and wellbeing. Work collaboratively with your health or social care colleagues at all times, such as when completing continuing healthcare checklists for safe discharge from hospital.
- *Information, advice and advocacy* – this theme concerns supporting people to make informed choices about their care and support, and its funding. This includes signposting to other services and promotes wellbeing through increasing a person's ability to make choices and take control.
- *Safeguarding* – safeguarding boards are set up in all areas to support people at risk of abuse and neglect. Everyone working in health and social care has a duty to report signs of abuse and neglect. Local safeguarding boards have websites with resources for professionals (please look up your local board's website as these are area specific).

RESOURCES

RCOT has published a series of booklets, *Care Act 2014: Guidance for Occupational Therapists*, available from www.rcot.co.uk. I advise you to read these as the information and guidance are invaluable. Another useful resource is Department of Health (2014) *The Care Act: Easy Read Version.* Newmarket: Inspired Services. Available from www.disability.co.uk/sites/default/files/resources/Making_Sure_the_Care_Act_Works_EASY_READ.pdf).

Mental Capacity Act 2005

This Act came into force in April 2005 and provides a framework for acting and making decisions on behalf of adults who lack capacity to make decisions for themselves. Believe it or not, the Mental Capacity Act (MCA) makes for an interesting read. It is particularly important for occupational therapists as it covers all areas of practice and at some point in your career you will be expected to carry out a mental capacity assessment with a person identified as needing care and support:

- on a hospital ward when making a decision about discharge
- undergoing rehabilitation in an intermediate care setting
- in a care home making decisions on returning to independent living
- in their own home when making a decision about equipment
- when considering manual handling to ensure safe transfers.

The list could go on for several pages; essentially it relates to *choice and control* around decisions and/or permission for interventions. Make sure you have the appropriate training before engaging in this assessment. That said, it is useful to sit in (with permission) and observe the assessment process. It is to be hoped you will have had this opportunity while on practice placement.

The first principle of the act is that we always assume a person has capacity *unless* it is established they do not. There needs to be proof their capacity is in question, for example brain injury, confirmed diagnosis of a mental condition, stroke, etc. All practical steps to support decision-making need to be evidenced as having been unsuccessful. (Make friends with speech and language therapists for this part, or use images/pictures to facilitate decision-making.)

Any decisions made for a person under the MCA must be done in their *best interest* and not led by other people's agendas, for example family, carer, doctor, etc. Before making a decision or undertaking an intervention consider if it is the least restrictive option available. Ask yourself if the decision or intervention will deprive the person of their liberty; is it excessive control?

> Remember, just because a person makes an unwise choice it does not mean they lack capacity.

This Act does not provide a broad-brush approach – you will be completing individual assessments in relation to decisions or actions at a given time. Being asked to complete a mental capacity assessment with a patient without a clear idea of what is being assessed should be challenged. If the answer is 'Oh, life in general', then where do you start with that? It simply can't be done. It is important to have a good understanding or knowledge of the person you are completing the assessment on. If you are unsure, ask for help from a person who has been working with them. You should consider the following:

- When are they at their best? – Choose a time of the day when they are least tired or most lucid.
- Can they hear/understand? – Is there somewhere to complete the assessment where it is quiet? Do they need an interpreter or new batteries for their hearing aid? What is the best method of communication?
- Do they need an advocate? – An independent mental capacity advocate (IMCA) will offer the support needed to ensure the person's best interest is at the heart of the assessment.
- What are the least restrictive/invasive options for this person?

If at any point you are unsure about completing the assessment, then ask or defer to another professional with appropriate training. It is essential you understand the implication of your role when decision-making with others. The MCA has been put in place to protect the most vulnerable people in our communities – remember this at all times.

Housing Grants, Construction and Regeneration Act 1996

Detail on this act is to be found in Chapter 10, 'Adaptations'.

Lifting Operations and Lifting Equipment Regulations (LOLER) 1998

LOLER came into force in December 1998 aiming to reduce risks to health and safety from lifting and it applies to equipment provided for use at work. These regulations require equipment to be strong and stable enough for use with the intended load (which applies to people as well as inanimate loads) and all lifting equipment must be marked indicating the safe working load. This includes accessories such as slings, for example, these must also be visibly marked with appropriate information for safe usage.

It is not only equipment which is covered by LOLER. To ensure safe use, LOLER requires equipment's use to be organised, planned and executed by competent people and that a regime is in place for ongoing examination and inspection by competent people

Hoists, slings and bath hoists are covered by these regulations, which state lifting equipment should be thoroughly examined by competent people at least every six months in the case of equipment used to lift people and at least annually in the case of other equipment.

It is important to know what duty you have to carers to make sure the environment you are designing meets their needs as well as the clients.

Provision and Use of Work Equipment Regulations (PUWER) 1998

PUWER came into force in December 1998 and places a duty on people and companies that own, operate or have control over work equipment. It requires equipment provided for use at work is suitable and safe for its intended use, maintained and inspected to ensure it does not deteriorate and become unsafe and used only by people who have received adequate training and information.

PUWER also stipulates equipment for work use is accompanied by suitable health and safety measures, such as protective devices and controls (emergency stop devices) and that equipment is used in accordance with specific requirements.

For occupational therapy this legislation is particularly important in relation to moving and handling equipment and should be incorporated in your manual handling assessments. Please read Chapter 11 on this subject. You will also need to read and act on any medical devices alerts relating to equipment used for work. Misuse of or incorrect guidance in the use of equipment for work can, and has, resulted in allied health professionals being prosecuted and losing their registration.

Community Care (Delayed Discharges etc.) Act 2003

Part 2 of this Act provides that any community care equipment and minor adaptations for the purpose of assisting with nursing at home or aiding daily living should be provided free of charge, providing the cost is £1000 or less. It requires local authorities to make payments to NHS bodies where a person's discharge from hospital is delayed because care services or services to carers have not been provided. Equally it also requires NHS hospitals to notify local authorities of anyone who is likely to need community care services when they are discharged from hospital.

Equality Act 2010

The Disability Discrimination Act has been incorporated into the Equality Act. The definition of disability contained within the Equality Act is crucially linked to a person's *ability to carry out activities of daily living* rather than simply to their condition or impairment, that is 'a disabled person is someone who has a physical or mental impairment that has a substantial and long term adverse effect on his or her ability to carry out normal day to day activities' (Equality Act 2010). The definition of disability includes those with cognitive impairments such as autism. When considering people who rent their home, there is a duty for landlords to not withhold consent unreasonably for 'adjustments' or adaptations.

Better Care Fund 2013/14

This promotes pooling of resources between health and social care services. The DFG is largely unaffected, although allocation of monies is now through/via the Better Care Fund. The changes arising from this act are still evolving so liaising with colleagues and keeping up to date are needed.

Chronically Sick and Disabled Persons (CSDP) Act 1970

Provision for assessing needs of people with disabilities is contained in the CSDP Act. The provisions are wide ranging and include an assessment for adaptations to the home or equipment for greater safety, ease or convenience. The Act requires local authorities to inform themselves of the numbers and needs of disabled people in their areas.

Section 2 lays out a range of services, including assistance with home adaptations, or the provision of any additional facilities designed to secure greater safety, comfort or convenience, which authorities should provide.

Children must be defined as disabled within the meaning of Section 17 of the Children Act 1989, and a child must be ordinarily resident within the area of the local authority. Top-ups for grants can be provided under this Act, though legally a local authority can restrict provision due to resources. Children's services authorities therefore have responsibilities for ensuring that assessments of needs, which might best be met by the provision of equipment and/or adaptations are carried out under the CSDP Act.

The CSDP Act is amended by the Care Act 2014 in respect of certain provisions that apply to adults in England while ensuring the provisions continue to apply in Wales. If you are unsure of a 'particular' provision that you have in mind check the legislation.

UN Convention on the Rights of the Child 1989

The convention came to force in the UK in 1992 and has 54 articles covering all aspects of a child's life. The convention must be seen as a whole as all the rights link and dovetail, creating an overall picture explaining how adults and governments must work together to ensure children enjoy their rights. The articles particularly pertinent for occupational therapy are:

- Article 31 (Leisure, play and culture): Play is recognised as a fundamental human right. Children have the right to relax and play, and to join in a wide range of cultural, artistic and other recreational activities.
- Article 23 (Children with disabilities): Children who have any kind of disability have the right to special care and support, as well as all the rights in the Convention, so that they can live full and independent lives.

Take time to read the summary of the convention on the United Nations Children's Fund (UNICEF) website (www.unicef.org.uk).

Children Act 1989

The Children Act became law in October 1991, requiring local authorities to provide a range of family support services for children in need. The definition of 'children in need' includes disabled children. Local authorities have specific duties to disabled children and their families, which require them to maintain a register of disabled children, provide services to minimise the effect of disabilities and enable them to lead normal lives. Occupational therapy assessments under the Children Act should be undertaken in conjunction with assessments under the Chronically Sick and Disabled Person's Act.

- Schedule 2 to the Act requires that local authorities provide services to minimise the effect on disabled children of their disabilities and give such children the opportunity to lead lives, which are as normal as possible.
- Section 17 imposes a target duty upon local authorities to safeguard and promote the welfare of children in their area who are in need by providing a range and level of services appropriate to the child's needs. It is not a specific duty to an individual child.
- Section 23 states the local authority has a duty to provide accommodation for a child in local authority care and to maintain that child. If the child is disabled, it is their duty to ensure accommodation is not unsuitable for that child.

Human Rights Act 1998

This Act came into force in October 2000 and covers a wide range of rights that not all countries, cultures and religious bodies agree with. The most prominent rights to consider are:

- *fundamental rights* – to live, be a citizen, to housing and to own property
- *safety* – to be safe from violence, seek asylum, have a fair trial and to be considered innocent until proven guilty
- *life freedoms* – right to an education, to healthcare, to believe and practise the religion a person wants.

- *sexuality and procreation* – right to marriage, equality of sexes, expression of sexual orientation, not be forced into marriage
- *political freedom* – free speech, right to vote, peacefully protest and to petition.

Along with these rights come responsibilities: consideration of others and the understanding that each person is an individual with their own sense of purpose and will.

Autism Act 2009

The Act came into force in January 2010 and makes provision about the needs of adults who have autism. (Children with autism are covered by the Children Act 1989.) Autism is a complex condition with a myriad of connecting presentations. Adults with autism have experienced, and still do experience, difficulties accessing services as they may not be diagnosed correctly or 'fall between' mental health and learning disabilities. The Act places the onus on NHS and local authorities to provide:

- relevant services for diagnosing autistic spectrum disorders (ASD) in adults
- identification of adults with ASD
- assessment of need for relevant services
- planning for the provision of relevant services during the transition period between child and adult
- training of staff who work with and/or provide services to adults with ASD.

Diagnosis is key to ensuring adults with autism receive support and services they need. It is important to note there are degrees to autistic traits, from low functioning to high functioning. It will be dependent on your skill as an occupational therapist to pick up on these and provide appropriate signposting to specialist services as required. If you have not had a learning opportunity already, ask for training on autism, or seek out alternative training opportunities as part of your continuing professional development (CPD).

Freedom of Information (FOI) Act 2000

The full provisions of this Act came into force on 1 January 2005 after much political wrangling and amendments. It is without question that you *must* have training on this legislation as it has implications on your recording and sharing of information. The Act applies to all public authorities in the UK, that is NHS, schools, universities, local authorities etc. and creates a general right of access, on request, to information these public authorities hold.

On receipt of an FOI claim a public authority has two corresponding duties. First (under s1(1)(a)) a duty to inform whether or not it holds the information requested and, second, if it does hold this information, to communicate it to the person making the request (s1(1)(b)). This is further supplemented by an additional duty to aid individuals in making requests and ensuring they frame their FOI requests appropriately (s16(1)).

In general, public authorities have 20 working days to respond to an information request, though this deadline can be extended in certain cases and/or with the agreement of the requester. Under the Act public authorities are encouraged to enter into a dialogue with the requester to better determine the information they want and the format they want it in.

Your place of work will have policies and procedures relating to this Act. You must read the policy and follow all procedures appropriately. Always check with your line manager if you are ever unsure about your recording and storing of information. Any public authority which comes under this piece of legislation will have an allocated FOI officer or office (team of workers) who will also be able to provide you with support and direction on the procedures or course of action. The Royal College of Occupational Therapists (RCOT) has excellent resources on this subject; make good use of them.

Data Protection Act 1998

This Act came into force in March 2000 and relates to the protection of personal data stored on computers and paper filing systems. It does not apply to information for domestic use such as address books. The Act controls how personal information is used by organisations, businesses and governments.

You, and anyone responsible for using data, have to follow the 'data protection principles' to make sure the information you keep is:

- used fairly and lawfully
- used for limited, specifically stated purposes
- used in a way that is relevant and not excessive
- accurate
- kept for no longer than necessary
- handled according to people's data protection rights
- kept safe and secure
- not transferred out of the European Economic Area.

Think about the work diaries you keep (paper and electronic), what would happen if they were inappropriately accessed by others? Anonymise or use initials when making appointments. Store your work/appointments diary carefully and report any data protection breaches as soon as you are aware they have happened.

Think about your recording of information and apply the data protection principles to this. Ensure your recording is appropriate, relevant and a true reflection of what has happened. Some workplaces will have specific ways of recording information; these will be laid out in the policies and procedures relating to data protection information. It is imperative you complete all compulsory training relating to this legislation as part of your induction.

> **NOTE**
> This act is to be replaced by the EU General Data Protection Regulation (GDPR) on 25 May 2018, becoming the Data Protection Act 2018.

Final words

The legislation in this chapter has been touched on briefly with the purpose of providing you with a basic understanding or 'taster' of core Acts providing a legal framework to why and how we do what we do. There will be an expectation for you to have knowledge of legislation and thus we urge you to make best use of all the resources available to you prior to the start of your working life. As you can see, there are amendments to all Acts and, as politics change, so it follows will legislation.

Once you are in the workplace, there will be pressures on you to concentrate on your case and workloads. (To be fair, it is easy to fall into a routine of concentrating on your caseload.) Remember part of the workload associated with cases will relate to legislation, thus it is imperative you keep up to date with any changes, either through training or as part of your CPD. Legislation is put in place to protect the most vulnerable in our society and to promote the rights and responsibilities of individuals, private agencies, public authorities and, of course, you yourself.

Be proactive, work with legislation, allow it to be a friend and let it work with you.

13

THOUGHTS ON INFORMATION GOVERNANCE AND DATA PROTECTION

Ruth Parker and Julia Badger

We are all aware of these obligations and frameworks, I can sense pages being turned, looking for 'more important' information. *Hold on a moment, indulge us!* We are not going to bore you with detail but to set them in the big picture of your working world.

First, a quick word of warning – as this book goes to print there is a major change – from 25 May 2018 the Data Protection Act (DPA) 1998 is no longer the relevant act – the General Data Protection Regulation (GDPR) will be adopted and after this date will be the **Data Protection Act 2018**. This reflects the digital world we live in and has a few key changes and is more robust. As we said, we aren't going to bore you with detail, just remember advice may not reflect the relevant act – so please check, and double check!

All large organisations (health trusts/local authorities) will have policies in place and teams to oversee both training (usually mandatory) and practice. Apart from this, how will it affect you?

Think of it in terms of your role, you will be a communicator and negotiator. These roles require you to share and receive information in many ways, maintaining the privacy and dignity of those you are working with. The modern world has given us many electronic tools to share information but, remember, speech and pen and paper are just as relevant.

We must record our interactions with patients/service users. This is set out in the Health and Care Professions Council (HCPC) and Royal College of Occupational Therapists (RCOT) guidelines and will be part of your employer's requirements. How we do this (professional language, relevance of information) is the first step, but following this what happens to this information? Are your handwritten notes added to a paper file, shredded or bundled in the back of a drawer? Is your PC/tablet locked when you step away? Don't forget your smartphone as well. We work in busy environments. On wards there will be changes of personnel, visitors and patients; in an office there may be cleaning staff, window cleaners or members of other services, none of whom need to know the information you are recording.

Let's start with conversations. Sometimes we are required to gather and pass on information in an area where others may overhear. Think about bedside conversations or those at the nurses' station. Who else is around? Can the conversation be held elsewhere? This is not only an issue on wards. Out-patients, occupational therapy departments, A&E, etc. may require some discretion. Passing conversations in more public areas, corridors, canteens, etc. may be opportunities in a busy day to catch up with colleagues but you have no awareness of others passing by who may be able to overhear.

Mobile phones mean we can communicate wherever we are – but it doesn't mean we should. This can be more of an issue for those working outside the NHS. There, whilst not ideal, those around you are usually part of the support network for patients but in social care this can be very different. In many areas there is a move towards 'agile working'. This is using 'touchdown' points – places where you can book a workspace away from your base. Here you will have no idea who your neighbours are at the desks around you. We can book in at schools, fire stations, children's centres etc., finding ourselves alongside representatives from Highways, Education and all the other aspects of local council provision. This isn't to say you shouldn't have conversations (on the phone or in person with co-workers) in these locations, work would be impossible! Just bear in mind the sensitivity and level of detail of information you are sharing, even though those around you are subject to the same restrictions and information governance guidelines.

Keeping any record up to date with personal information for an individual is key to minimise inappropriate information-sharing. If you are aware there has been a change of address or contact detail check and change the record if needs be. Take responsibility. You may prevent someone else passing on information which should not be shared.

The records we keep are not just for members of multi-disciplinary teams. Individuals can request their records – subject access requests (SAR). SARs can be made by, or on behalf, of an individual under Section 7 of the DPA 1998 but have to be written rather than verbal. If you receive one, this does not mean you immediately hand over everything. There will be teams who are responsible for managing SAR requests as there is data within records which isn't shared. Therefore, pass on any request as soon as possible, as there are timescales which must be met. If a request for records is made, it is ok to check they are up to date and to add recent notes or emails which may not yet be in place.

Freedom of information (FOI) requests are slightly different. These come under the Freedom of Information Act 2000, allowing anyone the right to request information held by public organisations. This does not apply to personal data (see above) but you may find you are asked to assist in providing data to respond to a request, such as how long waiting lists are, length of treatment regimes, staff sickness rates etc.

Information has to be shared. It is an essential part of what we do. A simple appointment letter can contain a wealth of information falling under the DPA 1998/2018. Getting the address right may appear to be basic but, all too often, people forget to update health and social care providers with new contact details.

If you are sending a letter or an email check the recipients. A couple of handy hints:

- If you arrange to share information with someone via email, ask them to email you first then save their email in your contacts. It is likely your email will follow a straightforward pattern such as 'initial.surname@organisation'. Whereas 'cutiepie227@...' may appear to be an easily repeated email address but was that two '2's or three? This principle works well for text messages also.
- If you are leaving a voice mail, don't go into too much detail. If a generic answerphone message is used, it may be sensible just to leave your name and contact details, asking them to call back. You cannot be certain whose phone you have reached. It is always better to be cautious.
- Disable auto-fill for email recipients. Yes, it is a pain searching for recipients but inadvertently sending an internal email

to the wrong 'Mary' is *still* a data breach, just as if they are external to your service.

Internal email systems within organisations are secure, as are embedded messaging systems such as within SystmOne. Then again, caution is no bad thing when considering information to include in the subject line. You may find there is already an established protocol in place. If not, use of initials, postcodes and NHS or other ID numbers limits the information which pops up on phones and laptop screens as an email appears in our ever-filling inboxes.

It is possible to set up secure email links to individuals or organisations or to email 'locked' files. Each organisation will have its policy on this so check first.

Standard versus secure email – hmm, now there is a dilemma. Setting up an appointment with someone outside your organisation, sharing an assessment, passing on a new contact number. Very easily done via email but are you passing information securely and in line with your organisation's guidelines and legislation? .GCSX and .NHS accounts are secure and support safe transfer of information – but to be 'secure' *both* accounts need to have the same high level of security.

Mistakes will be made; each organisation will have its own way of dealing with them. The best approach is to 'fess up' and rectify the error as soon as you realise. Much better than trying to ignore it. It won't go away and being proactive is better than being found out.

Scans and emails have pretty much replaced fax numbers but where there isn't a secure email address sending a fax may be the only way to share information. Check and double check the number (of course) and then check the receiving the fax machine is either in a secure area or that someone will be there to receive it. A call from them to confirm receipt assists in quieting the nagging doubt a fax machine may be sitting in a dusty corner of a room forgotten and unmonitored.

Back to agile working for a moment – it is great. *Be aware*, if you link to the local network for printing or scanning and don't update your settings, you are at risk of printing via a unit miles away and then desperately trying to find someone to ensure your document is dealt with appropriately.

The internet has changed so much and offers many opportunities and a fair few pitfalls. The Cloud supports communications outside intranets and local networks promoting links between organisations

– right? It's not that simple. Information sharing protocols need to be in place and adhered to even when the information isn't 'sensitive'. Your information governance team will be able to advise.

Now for social media, lifeblood for many who are connected 90 per cent of the time, no different to breathing in the hierarchy of importance. Teams often have Facebook and Twitter accounts and will have protocols (of course) attached to updating these. What about personal accounts? Being an occupational therapist and the amount of time you spend at work means for those who update accounts regularly there is every chance you will want to update friends, family and followers on aspects of your working life.

It is obvious you don't post identifying details of patients or service users. But what about an intervention which had an impact on you? Imagine you were in A&E or orthopaedics in the aftermath of a major incident, posting details of treatment for an unusual injury could mean others could identify the individual. How about supporting someone after a suicide attempt? Mentioning supporting someone for X number of weeks may seem an innocent remark, but again may enable others to put two and two together.

OK, so you don't post about treatments or patients – what about team members? Another minefield. If they are active on social media then they may be happy to be mentioned, their posts to be 'liked' or tagged in a photo. If not (and there are plenty who aren't) then asking before posting may assist in maintaining workplace relationships on an even keel. Sharing good news is lovely; engagements, babies, new jobs, but sometimes there is a difference between sharing within a small team and with the wider world.

The Caldicott Report (Department of Health 1997) established principles which are widely adopted and provide the necessary protection through a common-sense approach. If you work in an organisation which doesn't use these, then adopting them at a personal level wouldn't be a bad thing, especially if you are heading towards work in a role-emerging setting or in independent practice.

All is not doom and gloom – the majority of your working life you will share information safely, securely and using appropriate systems. Information governance is there to support you in being an effective practitioner, not to tie you in tangles of red tape and stop you in your tracks.

14

CLOSING THOUGHTS AND NEXT STEPS

Ruth Parker and Julia Badger

Thank you for sticking with us; if you have trawled through the whole book – congratulations! If you have picked out the parts you think are most relevant then we hope we have managed to enlighten you somewhat. Either way we hope our efforts have explained/clarified/taught you a little. If so, that is our hope and intention on starting out on this task achieved.

Learning linked to this book has been a two-way street, we have learned a lot, some linked to areas of practice we haven't experienced, some around legislation and good practice, but also how to write a book! We have also learned our friendship can stand the stresses of both working and writing together, not something either of us would ever have expected as we sat on opposite sides of an interview room way back in 2005.

The original germ of an idea grew and changed (for the better), and we appreciate the skills, knowledge and efforts of those who took up the challenge we proposed out of the blue. This book may have our names on the front cover but it is a collaboration – demonstrating one of the key themes across all the chapters, we don't work in isolation. Wherever we find ourselves as occupational therapists, we are working with others, be they our patients, service users, clients or members of a multi-disciplinary team. Reflecting back over the voices heard in this book, we have all emphasised the need to work with others to meet our goals. As you move forward into your career as an occupational therapist, remember this, as these people will be both support and inspiration as you progress, eventually finding yourself in this role for future graduates.

We mentioned 'voices'; we hope you will have heard our contributors' voices come through clearly. Each has taken a different route to where they are now, all at different stages of their careers. This isn't intended to be a book written by those closer to the end of their 'illustrious careers' imparting wisdom which 'must be heeded' to those setting out as occupational therapists. Definitely not! This is intended to be a resource to assist you in adjusting to the workplace – think of it as an additional team member, one with the time to sit and explain what it is like to be an occupational therapist at a time and place which suits you, away from the demands of work. (For Ruth, starting out at 21 straight after graduation with limited life experience, this book is 30+ years too late but would have been *such* a help!)

You are busy making choices which will shape your life – either through selection of a specialism or work location, moving on from life as a student. We too are taking our next steps. As the book is passed to the publishers Julia is moving on to her new role and Ruth working hard writing her thesis, we hope having a completed document as this is published. Then? Who knows? Whatever life brings we will continue to learn and develop, identifying our meaningful occupations – and enjoying them!

Wherever life takes you we wish you all the best – good luck!

References

Age UK (2017) *Later Life in the United Kingdom.* (Updated on a monthly basis.) Accessed on 29/11/2017 at https://www.ageuk.org.uk/globalassets/age-uk/documents/reports-and-publications/later_life_uk_factsheet.pdf?dtrk=true.

Alzheimer's Society (2017) *Learning Disability and Dementia.* Accessed on 29/11/2017 at www.alzheimers.org.uk/info/20007/types_of_dementia/37/learning_disabilities_and_dementia.

American Psychiatric Association (2013) *Diagnostic and Statistical Manual of Mental Disorders,* 5th edn. Washington, DC: American Psychiatric Association.

Ayres, A. (2005) *Sensory Integration and the Child,* 25th anniversary edn. Los Angeles: Western Psychological Services.

Baum, C. and Christiansen, C. (2005) 'Person-Environment-Occupation-Performance: An Occupation-Based Framework for Practice.' In C. Christiansen, C. Baum and J. Bass-Haugen (eds) *Occupational Therapy: Performance, Participation, Well-Being,* 3rd edn. Thorofare, NJ: SLACK Incorporated.

Berry, J. and Ryan, S. (2002) 'Frames of reference: Their use in paediatric occupational therapy.' *British Journal of Occupational Therapy 65,* 9, 420–426.

British Standards Institution (2018) *Design of an accessible and inclusive built environment. Buildings. Code of practice.* (BS 8300-2:2018). London: BSI.

Brookes, A. (2008) 'Manual handling questions.' *The Column 20,* 1, 11–13.

Case-Smith, J. and Clifford O'Brien, J. (2014) *Occupational Therapy for Children and Adolescents,* 7th edn. St Louis, MO: Elsevier Mosby.

Centre for Accessible Environment (2018) *Wheelchair Housing Guide.* Accessed on 29/01/2018 at http://cae.org.uk/resources/publications.

College of Occupational Therapists (2006) *Recovering Ordinary Lives: The Strategy for Occupational Therapy in Mental Health Services 2007–2017, A Vision for the Next Ten Years.* London: College of Occupational Therapists. Accessed on 29/11/2017 at www.rcot.co.uk/practice-resources/rcot-publications/downloads/rol-vision.

College of Occupational Therapists (2015) *Code of Ethics and Professional Conduct.* London: College of Occupational Therapists. Accessed on 29/11/2017 at www.rcot.co.uk/sites/default/files/CODE-OF-ETHICS-2015_0.pdf.

Cooper S., Smiley E., Morrison J., Williamson A. and Allan L. (2007) 'Mental ill health in adults with intellectual disability: Prevalence and associated factors.' *British Journal of Psychiatry 190,* 1, 27–35.

Cooper, S. and van der Speck, R. (2009) 'Epidemiology of mental ill health in adults with intellectual disabilities.' *Current Opinion in Psychiatry 22,* 5, 431–436.

Department of Health (1971) *Better Services for the Mentally Handicapped.* London: HMSO.

Department of Health (1997) *The Caldicott Committee Report on the Review of Patient-Identifiable Information.* Accessed on 29/11/2017 at http://webarchive.nationalarchives.gov.uk/20130124064947/http://www.dh.gov.uk/prod_consum_dh/groups/dh_digitalassets/@dh/@en/documents/digitalasset/dh_4068404.pdf.

Department of Health (2001) *Valuing People, A New Strategy for Learning Disability for the 21st Century: A White Paper.* London: HMSO.

Department of Health (2009) *Valuing People Now: A New Three-Year Strategy for Learning Disabilities.* London: DH Publications. Accessed on 29/11/2017 at http://webarchive.nationalarchives.gov.uk/20130105064234/http://www.dh.gov.uk/prod_consum_dh/groups/dh_digitalassets/documents/digitalasset/dh_093375.pdf.

Department of Health (2012) *Transforming Care: A National Response to Winterbourne View Hospital.* Accessed on 29/11/2017 at www.gov.uk/government/uploads/system/uploads/attachment_data/file/213215/final-report.pdf.

Department of Health (2014) *The Care Act. Easy Read Version.* Newmarket: Inspired Services.

Dwyer J. and Reep J. (2008) 'How occupational therapists assess adults with learning disabilities.' *Advances in Mental Health and Learning Disabilities 2*, 4, 9–14.

EU General Data Protection Regulation (GDPR) (2018) Accessed on 13/12/2017 at www.eugdpr.org.

Gibbs, G. (1988) *Learning by Doing: A Guide to Teaching and Learning Methods.* Oxford: Oxford Further Education Unit.

Goodman, J., Hurst, J. and Locke, C. (2009) *Occupational Therapy for People with Learning Disabilities.* London: Churchill Livingstone Elsevier.

Hardy S., Chaplin E. and Woodward P. (2007) *People with Intellectual Disabilities: Mental Health Nursing of Adults with Learning Disabilities.* London: Royal College of Nursing.

Health and Safety Executive (2003) *The Principles of Good Manual Handling: Achieving a Consensus.* Sudbury: HSE. Accessed on 29/11/2017 at www.hse.gov.uk/research/rrpdf/rr097.pdf.

Health and Safety Executive (2011) *Getting to Grips with Hoisting People.* Accessed on 29/11/2017 at www.hse.gov.uk/pubns/hsis3.pdf.

Health and Safety Executive (2012) *How the Lifting Operations and Lifting Equipment Regulations Apply to Health and Social Care.* Accessed on 29/11/2017 at www.hse.gov.uk/pubns/hsis4.pdf.

Health and Safety Executive (2016a) *Health and Safety at Work: Summary Statistics for Great Britain 2016.* London: HSE. Accessed on 29/11/2017 at www.hse.gov.uk/statistics/overall/hssh1516.pdf?pdf=hssh1516.

Health and Safety Executive (2016b) *Manual Handling Operations Regulations 1992: Guidance on Regulations,* 4th edn. London: HSE. Accessed on 29/11/2017 at www.hse.gov.uk/pUbns/priced/l23.pdf.

Heslop P., Blair P., Fleming P., Hoghton M., Marriott A. and Russ, L. (2013) *Confidential Inquiry into Premature Deaths of People with Learning Disabilities (CIPOLD).* Bristol: Norah Fry Research Centre.

Heywood, F. (2001) *Money Well Spent: The Effectiveness and Value of Housing Adaptations.* Bristol: Policy Press.

H M Government (1970) Chronically Sick and Disabled Persons Act 1970. London: Stationery Office. Accessed on 13/12/2017 at www.legislation.gov.uk/ukpga/1970/44/pdfs/ukpga_19700044_en.pdf.

H M Government (1974) Health and Safety at Work Act 1974. London: Stationery Office. Accessed on 13/12/2017 at www.legislation.gov.uk/ukpga/1974/37.

H M Government (1983) Mental Health Act 1983. London: Stationery Office. Accessed on 13/12/2017 at www.legislation.gov.uk/ukpga/1983/20/contents.

H M Government (1989) Children Act 1989. London: Stationery Office. Accessed on 13/12/2017 at www.legislation.gov.uk/ukpga/1989/41/contents/enacted.

H M Government (1990) National Health Service and Community Care Act 1990. London: Stationery Office. Accessed on 13/12/2017 at www.legislation.gov.uk/ukpga/1990/19/contents.

H M Government (1992) Manual Handling Operations Regulations 1992. London: Stationery Office. Accessed on 13/12/2017 at www.legislation.gov.uk/uksi/1992/2793/contents/made.

H M Government (1996) Housing Grants, Construction and Regeneration Act 1996. Norwich: Stationery Office. Accessed on 13/12/2017 at www.legislation.gov.uk/ukpga/1996/53/contents.

H M Government (1998) Data Protection Act 1998. Norwich: Stationery Office. Accessed on 13/12/2017 at www.legislation.gov.uk/ukpga/1998/29/contents.

H M Government (1998) Human Rights Act 1998. Norwich: Stationery Office. Accessed on 13/12/2017 at www.legislation.gov.uk/ukpga/1998/42/contents.

H M Government (1998) Lifting Operations and Lifting Equipment Regulations 1998, SI 2307. Norwich: Stationery Office. Accessed on 13/12/2017 at www.legislation.gov.uk/uksi/1998/2307/contents/made.

H M Government (1998) Provision and Use of Work Equipment Regulations 1998. Norwich: Stationery Office. Accessed on 13/12/2017 at www.legislation.gov.uk/uksi/1998/2306/contents/made.

H M Government (1999) Management of Health and Safety at Work Regulations 1999. Norwich: Stationery Office. Accessed on 13/12/2017 at www.legislation.gov.uk/uksi/1999/3242/contents/made.

H M Government (2000) Freedom of Information Act 2000. Norwich: Stationery Office. Accessed on 13/12/2017 at www.legislation.gov.uk/ukpga/2000/36/contents.

H M Government (2002) Regulatory Reform (Housing Assistance) (England and Wales) Order 2002. Norwich: Stationery Office. Accessed on 13/12/2017 at www.legislation.gov.uk/uksi/2002/1860/pdfs/uksi_20021860_en.pdf.

H M Government (2003) Community Care (Delayed Discharges etc.) Act 2003. Norwich: Stationery Office. Accessed on 13/12/2017 at www.legislation.gov.uk/ukpga/2003/5/contents.

H M Government (2005) Mental Capacity Act 2005. Norwich: Stationery Office. Accessed on 13/12/2017 at www.legislation.gov.uk/ukpga/2005/9/contents.

H M Government (2009) Autism Act 2009. Norwich: Stationery Office. Accessed on 13/12/2017 at www.legislation.gov.uk/ukpga/2009/15/contents.

H M Government (2010) Equality Act 2010. Norwich: Stationery Office. Accessed on 13/12/2017 at https://www.legislation.gov.uk/ukpga/2010/15/contents.

H M Government (2014) Care Act 2014. Norwich: Stationery Office. Accessed on 13/12/2017 at www.legislation.gov.uk/ukpga/2014/23/pdfs/ukpga_20140023_en.pdf.

H M Government (2014) Children and Families Act 2014. Norwich: Stationery Office. Accessed on 13/12/2017 at www.legislation.gov.uk/ukpga/2014/6/pdfs/ukpga_20140006_en.pdf.

H M Government (2015/16) The Building Regulations 2010: Access to and Use of Buildings: Approved Document M. Newcastle upon Tyne: NBS. Accessed on 29/11/2017 at www.gov.uk/government/uploads/system/uploads/attachment_data/file/540330/BR_PDF_AD_M1_2015_with_2016_amendments_V3.pdf.

Holland A.J., Hon, J., Huppert, F.A., Stevens, F. and Watson, P. (1998) 'Population based study of the prevalence and presentation of dementia in adults with Down's syndrome.' *British Journal of Psychiatry 172*, 493–498.

Home Adaptations Consortium (2013) *Delivering Housing Adaptations for Disabled People: A Detailed Guide to Related Legislation, Guidance and Good Practice.* Nottingham: Care & Repair.

*i*dapt (2017) *idapt Planner.* Accessed on 29/11/2017 at www.idapt-planning.co.uk/room_layout_planner/.

Kielhofner, G. (2008) *A Model of Human Occupation: Theory and Application.* Philadelphia, PA: Lippincott Williams and Wilkins.

Kottorp, A. (2008) 'The use of the Assessment of Motor and Process Skills (AMPS) in predicting need of assistance for adults with mental retardation.' *OTJR: Occupation, Participation and Health 28*, 2, 72–80.

Kramer, P. and Hinojosa, J. (eds) (2010) *Frames of Reference for Pediatric Occupational Therapy*, 3rd edn. Baltimore, MD: Lippincott Williams and Wilkins.

Lane, S. and Schaaf, R. (2010) 'Examining the neuroscience evidence for sensory driven neuroplasticity: Implications for sensory based occupational therapy for children and adolescents.' *American Journal of Occupational Therapy 64*, 3, 375–390.

Lillywhite, A. and Haines, D. (2010) *Occupational Therapy and People with Learning Disabilities: Findings from a Research Study.* London: College of Occupational Therapists, Specialist Section on People with a Learning Disability.

Mansell, J. (2010) 'Raising our sights: Services for adults with profound intellectual and multiple disabilities.' *Tizard Learning Disability Review 15*, 3, 5–12.

May-Benson, T. and Koomar, J. (2010) 'Systematic review of the research evidence examining the effectiveness of interventions using a sensory integrative approach for children.' *American Journal of Occupational Therapy 64*, 3, 403–414.

Mencap (2007) *Death by Indifference.* London: Mencap.

Mesa, S., Heron, P., Chard, G. and Rowe, J. (2014) 'Using the Assessment of Motor and Process Skills as part of the diagnostic process in an inner-city learning disability service.' *British Journal of Occupational Therapy 77*, 4, 170–173.

Michael, J. (2008) *Healthcare for All: Report of the Independent Inquiry into Access to Healthcare for People with Learning Disabilities.* Accessed on 29/11/2017 at http://webarchive.nationalarchives.gov.uk/20130107105354/http:/www.dh.gov.uk/prod_consum_dh/groups/dh_digitalassets/@dh/@en/documents/digitalasset/dh_106126.pdf.

Miller, L., Coll, J. and Schoen, S. (2007) 'A randomized controlled pilot study of the effectiveness of occupational therapy for children with sensory modulation disorder.' *American Journal of Occupational Therapy 61*, 2, 228–238.

National Audit Office (2016) *Discharging Older Patients from Hospital.* Accessed on 29/11/2017 at www.nao.org.uk/wp-content/uploads/2015/12/Discharging-older-patients-from-hospital.pdf.

National Learning Disabilities Professional Senate (2015) *Delivering Effective Specialist Community Learning Disabilities Health Team Support to People with Learning Disabilities and Their Families or Carers: A Briefing Paper.* Accessed on 29/11/2017 at national_ld_professional_senate_guidelines_for_cldt_specialist_health_services_final_3_march_2015.docx.

National Institute for Health and Clinical Excellence (2015) *Challenging Behaviour and Learning Disabilities: Prevention and Interventions for People with Learning Disabilities Whose Behaviour Challenges.* NICE guideline [NG11]. Accessed on 29/11/2017 at www.nice.org.uk/guidance/ng11/chapter/introduction.

National Institute for Health and Care Excellence (2017a) *Hip Fracture: Management.* Quality standard [CG124]. Accessed on 29/11/2017 at www.nice.org.uk/guidance/cg124.

National Institute for Health and Care Excellence (2017b) *Falls in Older People.* Quality standard [QS86]. Accessed on 29/11/2017 at www.nice.org.uk/guidance/qs86.

NHS England (2014) *Five Year Forward View.* Accessed on 29/11/2017 at www.england.nhs.uk/publication/nhs-five-year-forward-view.

NSPCC (2016) *Safeguarding Disabled Children in England.* Accessed on 29/11/2017 at www.nspcc.org.uk/globalassets/documents/research-reports/safeguarding-disabled-children-england.pdf.

Nygard, L., Bernspang, B., Fisher, A. and Winblad, B. (1994) 'Comparing motor and process ability of persons with suspected dementia in home and clinic settings.' *American Journal of Occupational Therapy 48*, 8, 689–696.

Parkinson, S., Forsyth, K. and Kielhofner, G. (2006) *A Users Manual for Model of Human Occupation Screening Tool.* Accessed on 13/12/2017 at www.cade.uic.edu/moho/pdf/MohostManual.pdf.

Pfeiffer, B., Koenig, K., Kinnealey, M., Sheppard, M. and Henderson, L. (2011) 'Effectiveness of sensory integration interventions in children with autism spectrum disorders: A pilot study.' *American Journal of Occupational Therapy 65*, 1, 76–85.

Pool, J. (2008) *The Pool Activity Level (PAL) Instrument for Occupational Profiling: A Practical Resource for Carers of People with Cognitive Impairment,* 3rd edn. London: Jessica Kingsley Publishers.

Russell, R. (2017) 'Quality: What are we missing in home modifications?' Paper presented at the Home Modifications Australia (MOD.A) National Conference.

Schaaf, C.R., Hunt, J. and Benevides, T. (2012) 'Occupational therapy using sensory integration to improve participation of a child with autism: A case report.' *American Journal of Occupational Therapy 66*, 5, 547–555.

Schaaf, R., Benevides, T., Mailloux, Z., Faller, P., *et al.* (2013) 'An intervention for sensory difficulties in children with autism: A randomized trial.' *Journal of Autism and Developmental Disorders 44*, 7, 1493–1506.

Smith, J. (ed.) (2005) *The Guide to the Handling of People,* 5th edn. London: BackCare.

Smith, J. (ed.) (2013) *The Guide to the Handling of People,* 6th edn. Sunbury-on-Thames: BackCare.

Smith Roley, S., Mailloux, Z., Parham, D., Schaaf, R., Lane, C. and Cermak, S. (2015) 'Sensory integration and praxis patterns in children with autism.' *American Journal of Occupational Therapy 69*, 1, 1–8.

Social Care Institute for Excellence (2009) 'Inter-professional and inter-agency collaboration.' *Workforce,* August. Accessed on 29/11/2017 at www.communitycare.co.uk/2009/08/03/interprofessional-and-inter-agency-collaboration.

Stancliffe, R., Harman, A., Toogood, S. and McVilly, K. (2007) 'Australian implementation and evaluation of active support.' *Journal of Applied Research in Intellectual Disabilities 30*, 3, 211–227.

Stevenson, A. (ed.) (2010) *Oxford Dictionary of English,* 3rd edn. Oxford: Oxford University Press.

Turpin, M. and Iwama, M. (2010) *Using Occupational Therapy Models.* St Louis, MO: Churchill Livingstone Elsevier.

United Nations (1989) Convention on the Rights of the Child. Accesed on 13/12/2017 at www.unicef.org.uk/wp-content/uploads/2010/05/UNCRC_united_nations_convention_on_the_rights_of_the_child.pdf.

World Federation of Occupational Therapists (2017) *Statement on Occupational Therapy.* Accessed on 29/11/2017 at www.wfot.org/Portals/0/PDF/STATEMENT%20ON%20OCCUPATIONAL%20THERAPY%20300811.pdf.

World Health Organization (1992) *The ICD-10 Classification of Mental and Behavioural Disorders: Clinical Descriptions and Diagnostic Guidelines.* Geneva: World Health Organization.

World Health Organization (2014) *Mental Health: A State of Wellbeing.* Accessed on 29/11/2017 at www.who.int/features/factfiles/mental_health/en.

Zwicker, J. and Harris, S. (2009) 'A reflection on motor learning theory in pediatric occupational therapy practice.' *Canadian Journal of Occupational Therapy 76,* 1, 29–37.

Index